"I am sure all those who read about your journey will be inspired by your courage and strength."

—Rick Hansen, co-author of *Man in Motion*

"Being a cancer survivor myself, I can partly understand what Andrew had to endure as a nine year old when his world was shattered by a rare form of cancer. But his jovial, happy-go-lucky attitude helped him tackle the challenge as a game, a game he was able to win with the help and mercy of God. Today Andrew is a very positive, successful entrepreneur. It's a joy to have him and his wife Ono as members at New Life Church. A very inspiring read."

—Pastor Elio Marrocco, Lead Pastor at NewLife Church
and author of *Che Vedi*

"Members like Andrew, who have persevered in the face of adversity and who work toward bettering the lives of others, embody what it means to be a TREB member."

—Tim Syrianos, Toronto Real Estate Board President,
2017/2018

"An inspiring, moving and courageous account that provides hope to others on their journey"

—Chris Kotsopoulos, CEO/Directeur general,
Children's Wish Foundation of Canada

"*Survivor* is the courageous story of an extraordinary boy named Andrew Mizzoni. Andrew embarked on a journey that no one could ever expect—one filled with fear and uncertainty—but also a journey filled with courage and hope."

—Marc Caira, Former President and CEO, Tim Hortons Inc.

"It's not often you come across a young athlete who displays such quiet grace and inner fortitude in the face of immense personal hardship."

—Marissa Stapley, *Toronto Sun*

"This lad's strength should be an inspiration to anyone four, five or six times his age with half the problems."

—John Gardner, President, Greater Toronto Hockey League

"Andrew's quiet determination has inspired countless other young athletes – with cancer and without."

—*Today's Parent Magazine*

"Incredible as it sounds, he continued to play hockey while he underwent chemotherapy and radiation treatment for cancer"

—Lois Kalchman, *Toronto Star*

"In my mind I will refer to you as a great Canadian."

—Lane MacAdam, Director General, Sport Canada

"A one-eyed goalie and cancer survivor who has inspired his team and his community."

—Matthew Sekeres, *Ottawa Citizen*

"Consider Andrew Mizzoni the little goalie that could."

—Todd Saelhof, *Ottawa Sun*

"Andrew Mizzoni's courageous and joyous life continues to inspire."

—Mariella Policheni, *Corriere Canadese*

To Ben,

SURVIVOR

Overcoming Childhood Cancer
through Faith, Family, and Sports

ANDREW MIZZONI

Printed in Canada
ISBN: 978-1-4866-1711-1

Word Alive Press
119 De Baets Street Winnipeg, MB R2J 3R9
www.wordalivepress.ca

WORD ALIVE
—P R E S S—

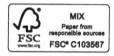

MIX
Paper from
responsible sources
FSC
www.fsc.org   FSC® C103567

Cataloguing in Publication information can be obtained from Library and Archives Canada.

For all those in the midst of their battle who line the halls and fill the beds of hospitals around the world.

Contents

Acknowledgements

To all those who played a part in my recovery: doctors, nurses, support staff, family and friends, my parents who were by my side every step of the way and my Lord and Saviour Jesus Christ, the mastermind behind my journey.

My beautiful wife, Ono, for her support, my dad for starting and documenting my journey, the team at Word Alive Press and all the contributors.

Foreword

Sometimes in life you come into contact with people who make a lasting impression on you. The Mizzoni family and their son Andrew made that type of impact on me and so many others.

I first met the Mizzoni family in the summer of 2013 when I was touring the country as the new Chief Executive Officer of Tim Hortons. Like many other franchisees, the Mizzonis were warm, proud and successful operators of their Timmies restaurants, located just north of Toronto. What I didn't know then—but would learn in subsequent months—was the tremendous battle, hardships and personal sacrifices they had made when their nine-year-old son was diagnosed with a rare form of cancer.

Survivor is the courageous story of an extraordinary boy named Andrew Mizzoni. Andrew embarked on a journey that no one could ever expect, one filled with fear and uncertainty, but also courage and hope.

This book teaches us the importance of never losing hope and of finding strength through family, friends and the community. Andrew Mizzoni's story shows us how to live true to your values and principles every single day and to fight through life's obstacles with an unrelenting and determined attitude.

Survivor is a remarkable story told through the lens of a nine-year-old who grows up to become the confident, loving and successful role model he is today.

Marc Caira
Former President and CEO
Tim Hortons Inc.

Introduction

This past week has been like none other I've lived through before. At only nine years old, I have just spent my last few days undergoing numerous procedures at SickKids Hospital in Toronto. The name of the hospital surely gives away the circumstances I'm in. The tests I've experienced for the first time involve scanning my entire body, including all my organs, bones, bone marrow, and even spinal fluid. I don't really know what to think. I go through the motions, from one room to the next, as they tell me it's what I have to do to get better, but so far the extent of my sickness is unknown. The doctors and nurses that cross my path say they can't believe how brave I am in dealing with the situation.

Now at the end of the week, I find myself in the waiting room of the Oncology Wing awaiting my test results. It's on the 8th and final floor of the hospital and, although I don't understand the meaning of "oncology," I know it isn't a pleasant word.

Throughout the day, this waiting room temporarily houses hundreds of children along with their families, but right now as the day draws to a close my parents and I are now the only people left in this room. We try to be patient as we await my results. My parents are exhausted and can't keep their eyes open any longer. They fall asleep on a long couch while I play my favourite baseball game on a gaming device my brother let me borrow. I pause and look through a window to the food court in the atrium below where cleaning staff are mopping floors and lifting chairs onto tables as they close down for the night.

Footsteps suddenly trigger my attention. I look up and see several people approaching. I quickly wake my parents as the group pulls up chairs to be seated across from us. My new oncologist, Dr. David Malkin, has arrived with his team. He calls my parents out of the waiting room to speak with them privately.

"We'll only be a few minutes," the doctor tells me.

I sit alone, returning to my video game while wondering, in the calmest of ways, what they could be discussing.

Ten long minutes later they all return. My parents seem more emotional than they were.

The doctor then begins to speak. The next sequence of words out of his mouth will change the course of my life forever.

ONE
Early Years

I came into this world on Thanksgiving Day— October 14, 1991— at Humber River Regional Hospital in Toronto, Ontario, Canada, weighing six pounds, six ounces. With a name like Mizzoni there is little guessing that my ancestors hailed from Italy. In fact both of my parents, Leonard and Rita Mizzoni, are second-generation Canadians. My mother's family comes from the southern region of Molise, and my father's family originates from Frosinone, Lazio. Both my parents come from fairly large families. My mom is the fifth of seven children and my dad is the eldest of four boys. My parents first met when my father was playing in a band that happened to be doing a concert at my mother's high school. Their eyes met while she was in the crowd and he was on stage, and from that point their relationship sparked. Dad tells me stories of how he used to pick Mom up from work at the local donut shop and how she used to ride her bike to meet him. After dating for several years, my parents tied the knot, with Dad reciting an original love song to Mom during their wedding banquet.

My dad went on to have much success in the music industry, as part of the '80s band Frozen Ghost. They went from recording in a home studio to being signed to a major North American record company. Their first album achieved gold status in Canada and they took to the road as an opening act for major headliner Howard Jones, touring across Canada and the United States and playing such venues as Madison Square Garden and the LA Forum. My dad was the lead saxophonist who also played keyboards and acoustic guitar, and performed backup vocals. In 1987 they were awarded Canada's most prestigious music award, a Juno, for the Most Promising Group of the Year.

My dad left the group around the time my brother Justin was born, and when I came into the world a few years later, my father was working in the vehicle fleet management business and my mother, a university graduate, was working in a bank part-time.

They named me Andrew John, but my father always nicknamed me his "joy." When I asked my mother where she got my first name from, she responded, "I've always liked that name." My middle name is my father's middle name, which is derived from his father's first name. I came to a deeper appreciation of my name when I heard a sermon about the apostle Andrew, who was the first person to follow Jesus, and who brought his brother along. The sermon said we should all seek to be "an Andrew," someone who does great things and seeks no credit for them.

My parents were devoted Catholics who instilled in us the importance of faith, as did my grandparents. I have a strange vivid memory of heaven from before I was born, of sitting at a table, and seeing at the other end of the table a man who I know is Jesus. I'm called to stand up and I know, without words, that I need to leave this place, but that I will one day return.

As a small child, I was very quiet and barely spoke until the age of two, relying on my older brother Justin to speak and interpret for me. My mother brought me to see several specialists including a pediatric speech pathologist, but they all concurred that I was fine and that one day I would begin speaking and wouldn't stop. Boy, were they ever right! I became the child asking my parents questions about whatever topic came to mind. Still, today I tend to remain quiet until I feel comfortable around people and then I ask lots of questions.

My family lived in a cute three-bedroom home on a corner lot in Brampton, a large city northwest of Toronto. It was at this house that I had some memorable moments like trying to ride a bike for the first time, before falling down. I learned how to skate and rollerblade. Thankfully, my dad bought me kneepads and elbow pads. He used to take us to Gage Park in downtown Brampton to skate around to the sound of music, the sight of Christmas lights, and the delicious taste of hot chocolate. My mom, on the other hand, would take my brother and I to the nearby Chinguacousy Park to swim in the public pool.

When my dad came home from work, my mom would then start her shift at the local bank. My dad would cook us dinner, which was usually macaroni and cheese with hot dogs, or fish sticks, then the three of us would watch television together. Afterward, we would ride our bikes to visit my mom at work and be treated with a Dairy Queen peanut buster parfait which we would split three ways. Some evenings, Justin and I would play outside with friends until it got dark and the street lights came on. That was our cue to head home. One night a week my dad and I would escape to his room to watch another great show, "The X-Files" starring David Duchovny as Mulder. My brother was so scared of the show that he would run out of the room if it was on.

When I was eight years old, my family decided to pick up and move to Woodbridge, which is part of the City of Vaughan. When the construction of our new home was delayed, we moved in with my dad's parents to bridge the gap. I am very close with my grandparents. They also happened to live on a large lot where we could play golf, basketball, tennis, and anything else kids could find to amuse themselves with. To make things better than they already were, my Nonna is the greatest cook in the world, and would spoil us with our favourites.

My brother and I started the school year at a school named Our Lady of Fatima but halfway through the year, the wing of the school that my class was in was tested positive for mould. This caused us to complete the rest of our year at a different school. My class was assigned to a school called St. Margaret Mary, which was going to be my school when we moved into our new home. Every day, I would take the bus to Our Lady of Fatima and then from there get bussed to St. Margaret Mary.

Our new home was a four-bedroom house to accommodate our family which had now grown larger with the arrival of my brother Lenny. It was a beautiful home situated on a quiet court. I had a very nice room which overlooked the backyard. Our house was within walking distance of a community centre which was great. Even better was that two of my cousins around my age had moved into the area with their families.

My brother Justin and I quickly became friends with everyone in the neighbourhood. On my first day of school, I remember walking into Mrs. Arruda's class and sitting on the carpet. To my side was my soon to be good friend, Dean Dolcetti, who looked at my new Nike shoes and commented, "I like your shoes." As kids, it's very easy to meet new friends if you are open to the opportunity. Unlike our former home in Brampton, our new home was in an Italian-dominated community. We would often spend time together at the park or at the local community centre.

I was very young when my parents enrolled me in soccer and hockey in the community. I enjoyed both sports but my passion was being on the ice. (I actually still get made fun of by my parents for picking grass and staring at the sky during my first experience as a soccer goalie. I'm afraid that was the highlight of my illustrious soccer career.) Meanwhile, my hockey career began to take flight. During my first season in house league, I was given the opportunity to put on the goalie pads and play goal. I enjoyed it so much and was so good at it that I was quickly made the permanent goalie for my team. My family has a history of goalies with my dad's brothers Danny and Tommy both playing goal. The following season I took my team to the finals.

That next summer, I was so dedicated to improving that my dad took me to receive professional training. We went to Franco Canadian Goalie School, which was highly intensive training where we were trained heavily by experienced goalies, as well as getting to stop pucks from great players. I was probably the youngest goalie on the ice. After each session, I was drenched with sweat, but as the famous adage says:

"No pain, no gain." That fall, the gain arrived when my dad took me to a AA-tryout for our local team, the Vaughan Rangers. It was the second highest league in Canada for my age group. I showed off my skills in great fashion with my dad looking on proudly. After the tryout, we all waited to find out if we made the roster. When we were called in, Dad and I had very little expectations as we sat across from the panel of coaches. To our surprise, they said, "We want Andrew on our team." We graciously accepted the offer.

That season kept my family and me very busy at least four days a week, with a myriad of games, practices, and tournaments, but I loved it. I had such dedication that I never missed one practice or game and was always the first player on my team in the dressing room. I was also adamant on dressing myself in my goaltender equipment, while my peers all had to seek their parent's assistance. I think it was through hockey, as well as having an older brother close in age, that my competitive nature was born. I always wanted to play against the elite teams in the league and absolutely despised losing (a quality I still have to this day). But I did understand that you learn more from your defeats than your successes so after every loss, I'd grab a tennis ball and throw it off the wall and catch it in my glove or block it with my blocker for hours in my goalie stances. I was surely on my way to great success.

TWO
The Diagnosis

It was a Saturday morning in late March 2001 and I was nine years old. I vividly remember getting up that particular morning and walking down the stairs to eat breakfast like I always did, although this time I didn't race as I usually did, but went slowly and leaned on the banister, seeing my mother below eating her breakfast. My mother was eating the same thing for breakfast that she always has: a bowl of Kellogg's Raisin Bran cereal. (She eats so much of it that you'd think she owned shares in the company!) I reached the bottom of the stairs, stepped onto our green ceramic floor and walked past our hallway mirror toward the kitchen table.

"Stop!" my mother said. "Let me see your eye, Andrew." Noticing a slight difference in my eye, she asked me if perhaps I had hit it accidentally or had slept strangely. I didn't remember hitting it and I walked back to the mirror to see if I saw what she could. I did, in fact, notice a slight bulging under my left eye.

Curious to see whether this was worrisome or not, my mother arranged an appointment with our long-time family physician, Dr. Klar.

He wasn't too concerned when he examined me, but he did set up an appointment to see Dr. Kravetz, an ophthalmologist at Etobicoke General Hospital, After a thorough examination, Dr. Kravetz commented, "I'm not too concerned, but I will book a CAT scan for you just to make sure it's nothing."

The great thing about living in Canada is that health care is provided free of charge to residents; the downside is that the wait time to receive a treatment may take months before you can get in. My particular CAT scan was scheduled in six months. In the meantime, we would wait patiently and keep surveying my eye for any changes.

But only a few days after walking out of Dr. Kravetz's office, we began to notice that the swollen area under my eye was becoming hard. To the touch, it felt as if there was definitely something there that shouldn't be. To make matters worse, my left eye appeared to be off-centre and bulging. My mother quickly called Dr. Kravetz's office. The doctor's staff tried to dismiss my mother by stating that there was a scan already booked. But my mother can be very tough at times and is someone you want to have fighting in your corner. She persisted and demanded that I see the doctor right away. Her persistence paid off as she got me in to see Dr. Kravetz again that very day. While she, my dad and I sat in his waiting room, my mom struck up a conversation with one of the doctor's administrative assistants. My mom told her what had occurred in the last few days, and the lady responded: "If he was my son I would take him right down to SickKids Hospital." Standing nearby and minding my own business, I heard the words "sick kids" uttered for the first time about me. I had heard about this hospital before, a magical place where sick children could go to be made well again, but that's as far as my knowledge went. After Dr. Kravetz's second examination, he, too, was very concerned. He was so concerned that he moved up my CAT scan appointment to that afternoon.

We walked across the street to an alternate wing of Etobicoke General Hospital. My mom had to go home and take care of my siblings, while my dad and I remained. We waited for several long hours, until we were the only ones left in the large waiting room. We occupied the time by walking up and down the halls and sitting in various seats in the waiting room. I remember walking laps past a vending machine and glancing in to see what snacks were available. Finally, a nurse in a white lab coat called out, "Mizzoni, Andrew."

I followed her toward large doors with a flashing red sign that read "X-ray in progress." I didn't really know where I was going or even what a "cat scan" was. All I knew was that I had never really liked cats. A CAT scan, more properly known as a CT scan, stands for Computerized Tomography, formerly known as Computerized Axial Tomography. It's an x-ray procedure which generates cross-sectional views of the internal organs and structures of the body.

I was led into a large room with a flat table attached to a big donut-like shaped device in the centre of the room. I was told by the technicians in the room to lay down on the table, and my head was affixed in a particular position and held into place by soft sponge-like items on each side, along with a strap across the top. The technicians told me, "Try not to move and just relax; it'll be over before you know it." The technicians then left the room and, before I knew it, the bed slid inside the donut device and began to operate. I noticed the camera began to spin around my head, while a few stickers above my head caught my attention. Halfway through the process, a technician temporarily stopped the scan to inject me with a dye which allowed them to receive even better images. The dye was iodine containing contrast material and was put into the veins in my arm followed by a saline solution. The bed then slid back into the scanner to begin the second round of images. Through it all, I remained very calm and comfortable and may have even dozed off briefly.

Once the scan was complete we returned to the waiting room, waiting for Dr. Kravetz to arrive to review the results. To pass the time, I continued walking up and down the halls again in exploration. Finally, Dr. Kravetz came out with my test results. After reviewing them, he looked very concerned, and for the first time my name and the word cancer were mentioned in the same breath. He said, "This could be very serious. A representative from SickKids Hospital will be contacting you tomorrow to arrange for you to see an ophthalmologist there." True to his word, my parents received a call the very next day for an immediate appointment to visit a Dr. Pashby at SickKids Hospital.

The Hospital for Sick Children in Toronto is world-renowned for the work they perform with children. Its roots go back to 1875, when a group of women led by Elizabeth McMaster rented an eleven-room apartment, set up six cots and declared it to be a hospital for the treatment and admission of sick children. Over one hundred years later, each year, The Hospital for Sick Children, also known as SickKids Hospital, has approximately 15,000 children who stay in nearly 400 beds; almost 300,000 visits are made to more than 100 clinics; emergency staff treat 50,000 children; and 13,000 operations are performed. From the moment I took my first step into the hospital I was amazed. It was like nothing I'd ever seen before. As I entered into the open concept atrium, to my left, I saw large fountains pouring with water, to my right and above were an enormous toy clown and an elephant levitating in the air on a wire. We then passed by a gift shop full of fun stuff and a daycare area, following multi-coloured footsteps lining the halls. It was easy to see that this was a place for children.

We were there to see Dr. Pashby who turned out to be a great man with a very good bedside manner. During his careful observation of my eye, we spoke much about sports, especially hockey. Before making his diagnosis, Dr. Pashby wanted the top ophthalmologist in the city, Dr. Jeffrey Hurwitz, to give us a second opinion. On our way out of Dr. Pashby's office, my dad and I noticed a hockey helmet on his desk. Curiously I asked, "Why do you have a hockey helmet?" He went on to explain that his father, Dr. Tom Pashby, was the ophthalmologist who had helped develop the face mask, visor and helmet that all hockey players wear today. He had been inspired after his son who came home one day with a concussion he received while playing in a house league hockey game. I thought this was a very cool story and made me further like and feel comfortable with Dr. Pashby.

The next day, we went to visit Dr. Hurwitz first thing in the morning. Dr. Hurwitz's office was in Mount Sinai Hospital, across from SickKids Hospital on University Avenue. We rode up the main escalators to his clinic with much anticipation. On the walls of his office were plenty of sports memorabilia, including one image of the Toronto Maple Leafs dressing room with one jersey bearing the name Hurwitz on the back. My dad and I glanced at each other, as this sign was reassuring. While Dad signed me in, I began reading a *Sports Illustrated* magazine. Minutes later we were called into one of two rooms. As my dad and I sat there, we wondered what Dr. Hurwitz was like, as we looked in awe at all the prestigious plaques he had on his wall.

He turned out to be unlike most doctors, entering the room by exuberantly saying, "Hey guys!" I immediately thought he was very cool and down to earth. We spoke about sports the entire time and I found out he was the eye doctor for the Toronto Raptors basketball team. He was also a season ticket holder of the Toronto Rock lacrosse team. After his analysis, he told us that in order to find out for sure what we were dealing with, I would have to have a biopsy. I had never heard that word before, so when asked by a family member what had happened at the hospital, I would respond: "I have to have an autopsy!" I guess I picked it up from my days of watching "The X-Files." My dad would quickly interject and say, "No, Andrew, you're having a biopsy; autopsies are for when people die." My autopsy—I mean, biopsy—was scheduled for that same Friday. Since Dr. Pashby was a registered surgeon at SickKids Hospital, he was going to perform the surgery, as he was able to gain access to an operating room sooner than Dr. Hurwitz could. He cancelled all his morning appointments in order to perform my biopsy.

On Friday morning, my family and I travelled down to SickKids to meet with Dr. Pashby prior to my surgery. He immediately noticed that the still unknown growth had grown considerably since he had last seen me, a week prior. While I was preoccupied playing my video game, Dr. Pashby looked at my parents in a very concerned way and said, "I suspect it is something sinister."

I then sat and waited in the waiting room. Upon a nurse calling my name. I got up, got weighed and height-tested and then changed behind a curtain into my hospital wear. The hospital gown consisted of loose pants that were tied by string and an upper body portion which was a little tricky to put on. I had to place my arms in first and then secure it with a knot on my back for which I needed help to complete. I then went back into the waiting room until an anesthesiologist came by to ask me several questions pertaining to allergies, as well as giving me my anesthetic flavour options. Of the options I chose orange, but they explained to me that for some strange reason, the orange anaesthetic often made others present in the room sick, so I settled for watermelon. Before long, I was called again to say my farewells to my family, and then was led into the operating room. I was amazed at all those who would be present and assisting with my biopsy. I hopped up onto the surgical table in the middle of the room and was connected with several devices including a blood pressure monitor on my finger. Then came the anesthetic administered through a gas mask which looked like something a jet pilot would wear. Now, I'd had my fair share of watermelons before, but this anesthetic did *not* taste like the watermelons I was used to. Within a minute, I started to feel the effects as I faded away slowly into the sounds of the equipment beeping in the room.

For my parents, awaiting the completion of my biopsy felt like a lifetime. During my recovery, Dr. Pashby attended to my parents in the waiting room, bringing them the results. He sat next to them and explained, "It *is* a tumour and it looks malignant, but I won't know for sure until the results of the biopsy are returned." The word 'malignant' refers to a tumour that may easily spread to other tissues in the body.

I recovered from the procedure with ease and later left for home with my parents. But every time the phone rang in our home, my parents would jump up to answer, thinking it could be the hospital calling. Three long days after my biopsy, the results were in.

Dr. Pashby called my dad on his cell phone with a call my dad later described as one no parent should ever have to receive. Dr. Pashby began by saying: "Andrew has a malignant tumour called rhabdomyosarcoma." He went on to explain that it was a very rare form of children's cancer, with only twenty cases a year found in Canada, usually in children between the ages of five and ten years old. He continued, "This type of cancer does spread to other parts of the body very rapidly, so the next step is to perform a variety of biopsies, x-rays and tests to confirm if the cancer has spread, and to what extent." My dad couldn't believe his ears that this was his nine- year-old son the doctor was talking about.

Feeling distraught after the phone call, my dad decided to leave his office and go outside for some fresh air. While outside, he couldn't help but let out a few tears of worry for his son and the battle he would soon face. When he went back into his office, he sat down at his computer and began researching the type of cancer. While doing so, he began to get very emotional, as the more information he found, the more stressed he became. My dad was always the first one into the office and one of the first to leave but that day he prolonged his stay at the office, fearing having to face his family with the bad news he had been given. While his colleagues had all left for the day, my dad remained. The owner of the company, John Carmichael, happened to be walking by and spotted my dad. He asked: "Hey Len, why are you still here?" My dad began to share with John the news he had received earlier that day. Feeling my dad's pain, John offered a few words of encouragement and then went back to his office to grab something. He came back a few minutes later to give my dad a special book called *Healing Promises*, written by Christian evangelists Kenneth and Gloria Copeland. We carried this book with us through every hospital visit in my "hospital backpack" which housed all the documents we received throughout my treatment and I still have

had the pleasure of meeting John Carmichael while attending work with my dad one day. He is a great man, a successful was so well-liked that he later became a Member of Parliament for Canada.

When Dad mustered up enough strength he returned home to share the results of the phone call from earlier that day with my mom. You can only imagine how the woman who gave birth to me must have taken the news. But my parents found it very difficult to break the news to me, so they decided to let the doctors explain it, hoping they would be able to do so in a way that I would be able to understand. But word of my condition quickly spread to my family and friends, and even though I didn't know it, they began praying for me during what happened to be the season of Easter, which celebrates the death and resurrection of Jesus.

Rhabdomyosarcoma is a highly malignant type of cancer. It often spreads to various parts of the body, most commonly the brain and the lungs. If it spreads to these areas of the body, the chances of survival are very poor. That was why I had to undergo tests immediately to determine the severity of the cancer and whether it was contained. I underwent another CT scan, this time at SickKids.

The experience was similar to the one at Etobicoke General Hospital, except I had to drink the dye instead of receiving it directly through my veins. It was mixed with apple juice and tasted absolutely disgusting, but I had to force two glasses down while attempting to plug my nose. Also, this time, my dad got to stay in the room with me as long as he wore a blue vest which protected him against radiation exposure. Next, I received a bone scan. This machine also included a flat table on which I lay while a large rectangular scanning portion lowered on top of me. My dad called it a "waffle scan." It injected a very small amount of radioactive material called a tracer into my body. The tracer travels through your blood to the bones and organs. As it wears off, it gives off a little bit of radiation. This radiation is detected by a camera that slowly scans your body. The camera takes pictures of how much tracer collects in the bones. An abnormal scan will show hot spots and/or cold spots as compared to surrounding bone. Hot spots are areas where there is an increased accumulation of the radioactive material. Cold spots are areas that have taken up less of the radioactive material. Any abnormal findings would be compared with other tests and be assessed by doctors.

Although I could understand how some people could get claustrophobic during the bone scan, I was very comfortable. They had offered me a choice of movies I could watch during a long portion of the scan I was on my side, and I got so into the movie (*Flubber*, starring Robin Williams) that I forgot all about the big scan on top of me. I was about halfway through the movie when the scan was complete. On one hand, I was happy the scan was over; on the other hand, the movie was getting really good and I wanted to see the rest.

Next, I underwent a surgical procedure called a bone marrow biopsy. It was performed in a room on the eighth floor of the hospital called "Cujo's Kids" which had been donated by the Toronto Maple Leafs goaltender Curtis Joseph, of whom I was a big fan. As I entered the room for the first time, I was amazed by the way it was painted: on each side of the room it looked like the Maple Leafs dressing room, including each player's jersey. On the far wall adjacent to the door was a portrait of the famous Don Cherry and Ron MacLean from Coaches Corner" on "Hockey Night in Canada."

The bone marrow biopsy was crucial to see if the cancer had spread to other parts of my body. It involved sticking a foot-long needle into my spine in order to extract a portion of bone marrow. I was so in awe of the room I was in that I forgot all about the large needle. My parents, on the other hand and to their regret, saw the entire thing. When the bone marrow biopsy was done, I was allowed to choose a toy from the big treasure chest painted in Maple Leafs colours. I was unsure of which one to choose as every toy looked like fun. This signaled the last of a week's worth of testing. We had to await the results.

THREE

It's Cancer

Cancer, the word often feared to be spoken, has occurred and been recognized as such for thousands of years. The oldest documented case was recorded on papyrus in ancient Egypt around 3000 B.C. It describes eight cases of tumours or ulcers of the breast that were removed by cauterization with a tool called the fire drill. The writing says about the disease: "There is no treatment."

Thousands of years later, in 2001, I felt a warm sensation come over me as my new oncologist, Dr. David Malkin, began to speak. The first words out of his mouth were: "Andrew, you're sick, but the medicine we are going to give you is going to make you better." He then went on to explain the good news that my family was praying for: "You are still in the early stages of rhabdo and the tests from this week have all come back negative." That meant my tumour had not spread and was contained in my orbital region, which is the bony socket in front of the skull that contains the eye.

Dr. Malkin continued, "You will be treated over approximately a year with chemotherapy, along with the possibility of radiation and surgery." The reassuring part of the news was that my oncologist was confident that I would beat this. Dr. Malkin then went on to discuss in further detail what I had and some of the side effects I might experience. He said, "Your hair will fall out, but more importantly you will get better." He then provided me with some kid-friendly literature and a child's book to help answer any questions I might have. I still have this book in my hospital backpack. Looking back today as an advocate for positive thinking, I am very appreciative for the attitude my medical team displayed in this most difficult moment. This positive reinforcement also aided in getting me back to good health again.

Since I had such a fast-growing tumour, my first chemotherapy session had to be scheduled for early the next morning. After our talks concluded with the medical staff, my parents and I rushed home to grab some of my belongings. We gathered our things, took a momentary load off our feet, and then turned around and headed right back downtown to the hospital.

The term 'chemotherapy' was coined in the early 1900s by Paul Ehrlich to refer to the use of chemicals to treat any disease. The first modern chemotherapy agent was an arsenic compound to treat syphilis. This was later followed by sulfa drugs and penicillin. The first form of medicine used to treat cancerous cells originated during World War II. Members of the navy who had been exposed to mustard gas were found to have toxic changes in the bone marrow cells that develop into blood cells. The US Army had been studying chemicals related to mustard gas to develop protective measures. They studied a compound called *nitrogen* mustard that was found to work against a cancer called lymphoma. This became the model for similar compounds called alkylating agents that killed cancer cells by damaging their DNA. The era of chemotherapy had begun.

My own chemotherapy era began on April 9, 2001 when I was admitted at the Hospital for Sick Children's 8th floor oncology department. We headed to the wing opposite the clinic where in-patient chemotherapy was administered. My dad had always been my biggest supporter and believer. I was his little goalie, as he often called me. Throughout my sports career he would take me early to practices and games and stay to watch every minute of my performance. He would even buy me a milkshake or chocolate bar as a pre-game snack to give me a boost of energy. My mom, on the other hand, was usually at home watching my brothers but she came to my games every chance she got. I would always know when she was in the arena because I could hear her yelling in a high-pitched tone, "Focus, Andrew!" or "Smother it!" I don't know what I would have done without such supportive parents in my hockey career, and now in my cancer journey.

My dad and I checked in at the large oval desk and immediately were brought to my own hospital bedroom. My hospital room, which I would soon get to know very well, contained a hospital bed on the right side of the room, along with lots of equipment surrounding it. On the left side of the wall was a small sink which doctors and nurses would often use to wash their hands prior to performing a procedure. Up high on the left side of the room was a ledge which housed a television. Continuing on the left side of the room was the bathroom door. To the far-right side of the room was a tan-coloured couch with three pull-out drawers underneath. This was where my dad would usually sleep. Next to my bed was a dark coloured jug with a handle. I asked my nurse, "What is that for?" She explained: "That's for going pee if you can't use the washroom." I thought to myself: *why would I not be able to use the washroom?* But I would soon understand how important it was. On the far end of the room was a window that looked out into the atrium of the hospital.

Although my doctors and parents told me I was sick, I still had never heard anyone say that I had cancer. So, while lying in my hospital room in preparation for chemotherapy, I asked my dad in a soft voice, "Daddy, do I have cancer?" He responded, "Yes, Andrew." Then he reiterated what my doctor had told me earlier, "But this medicine is going to make you better again." I responded by simply saying "Okay."

Cancer had never been prominent in my family. Other than hearing of a few great-great-uncles in the Mizzoni family passing away from cancer when middle-aged, I had really only known one cancer survivor. It was my dad's cousin whom I called Uncle Rick. In his teens he had been diagnosed with osteogenic sarcoma in his leg, the same cancer that Terry

Fox suffered from. After a protocol which contained chemotherapy and radiation, he had had his leg amputated. But he went on to live a healthy life: he has a beautiful family with two children and a very successful career as a real estate developer. Shortly after my diagnosis, Uncle Rick took me and my dad out for dinner to a restaurant called Baton Rouge. The ribs were delicious.

My very first chemotherapy session began at 4:30 a.m. I was to be given two types of chemotherapy medicines: ifosfamide and etoposide (UP-16). Ifosfamide's purpose was to kill cancer cells, while etoposide was also used to kill cancer cells, along with stopping them from dividing and creating new cells. As I lay in my bed hooked up to the intravenous through my hand, I began to wonder what chemo would look or feel like. A nurse then came into my room wearing radioactive-protective equipment. She connected a bag of clear liquid into my IV. The chemo immediately gave my body a cooling sensation as it made its way through my veins. Not long after, I had my first reaction to the chemotherapy: nausea and vomiting. I grabbed the first bowl-like item in sight and put it to use. This would mark the first of many bouts of vomiting. I was then prescribed ondansetron, a medicine used for the prevention of nausea and vomiting, although I don't think it worked very well. I was also given a medicine called mesna which was used to reduce the harmful effects of chemo on the bladder. To pass the time between vomiting, I would watch television. I would watch "SportsCenter" often, but my favourite show had to be "The Price is Right." I became so familiar with the show that I started to know all the models' names. I'd also play with my Sega handheld device or play cards with my dad who stayed by my side the duration of my days.

Fortunately, my dad's career allowed him the flexibility of working from anywhere, so he would bring his laptop and get work done while in my hospital room. There was also a shower for parents on the other side of the wing; he would sneak out to use it at night when I was asleep. The food that was offered contained a few choices for every meal. Now that I've visited other hospitals, I realize how good I had it. Pizza, grilled cheese, and chicken noodle soup were some of the main courses, which would be accompanied by Jell-O, and juice. But, due to my state, I had very little appetite. Whatever I was able to consume would only last minutes before being thrown up into the bowl next to me. My "pee jug" also got used regularly as I became too weak to stand and walk to the bathroom, and also because I was connected to various devices and an intravenous. When I wasn't able to use the jug myself, my dad would hold it for me and later dump the remains down the toilet. (He reminds me all the time what he did for me and that one day I'll have to return the favour. If that time does come, I think I'd rather hire a pretty young nurse to take care of him instead—that would be a win-win scenario.)

Throughout my first stay in the hospital, we were very impressed with the attitude of the nurses as we began to get to know them very well. They made it a habit to introduce themselves when they started their shift: "Hi, my name is Samantha and I will be your nurse this evening. If you need anything at all please ask." Alternatively, when they finished their shift they would stop by and say: "My shift is over for the night, but is there anything you need before I go?" I asked the nurses about my eventual hair loss. One nurse said, "You should cut it short so that it won't bother you as much when it starts to fall out." Another nurse commented, "Some dads also shave their heads so that they can look the same." Another nurse dampened my spirits by saying: "Your hair may even grow back curly." I said, "I hope not, because I wouldn't look good with curly hair."

Chemotherapy is given in four- and five-hour intervals. Upon the completion of the treatment, my body then had to be flushed intravenously with liquids to remove any leftover toxins. During this "flushing" phase I was allowed to leave my room and roam the halls. SickKids Hospital has several fun areas to help pass the time including Marnie's Lounge on the 4th floor, the Starlight Lounge on the 9th floor, and the Teen Lounge also on the 8th floor. I also enjoyed just sitting on one of the benches in the hallway and looking outside over Elm Street.

I had now completed my very first chemotherapy session and couldn't have been happier to return home and see my family whom I hadn't seen in three days. It was a sunny evening when my dad's car pulled up in the driveway. As I walked through the door, Dad yelled: "Andrew's home!" I immediately made my way into the family room and curled up on one of the couches near the television and felt amazing comfort. I was home sweet home.

That weekend we decided to take the advice of the nurse: my dad took out the shaver that I had bought him for Christmas one year earlier and began to shave my head. My family was shocked by my new appearance. I, on the other hand, thought the new hairstyle looked cool and felt nice.

The first few days after returning home from chemo weren't always the most joyous. The nausea and vomiting streak which I experienced in the hospital continued, even when my body had no food in it and even after my grandmother brought me her famous rice with chicken soup which I loved. I always had an empty bowl within arm's reach. This made it very difficult for me to regain my strength. It was also extremely challenging to drink the required amounts of fluid since I was inactive. My parents would force me to keep drinking to flush my system, and even had me take a large plastic cup filled with water to bed.

Approximately seven to ten days after each round of chemo, old blood cells die and your body replenishes itself with new blood cells. Chemo apparently can affect these new cells in various ways. If my red blood cell count dropped, I would feel tired and look pale. If my platelets decreased, then my blood would have a problem clotting if I were to bleed. Most importantly, if my white blood cells were too low, then even the bacteria on my body could infect me. Thus, I had to take a medicine called filgrastim (G-CSF) to assist my bone marrow in producing white blood cells. It was administered via a needle. For the first trial, a nurse from SickKids came to show how it worked. Going forward, my dad took over and would give me the medicine daily. When the medicine made its way into my body, it gave my bones a cold sensation which is hard to describe. After only five days, my blood counts were so good that we got the okay to discontinue the use of G-CSF.

During the time off after my first chemotherapy session, I began to experience a few other side effects. For a few days, I had a sore lower back. This was something the hospital wanted to look into further. Secondly, I experienced some double vision, but we were later assured that it was common and that in time it would pass. Thirdly, I had to put up with my parents asking me: "How do you feel, Andrew?" every five minutes. Looking back, I understand the severity of the situation we were going through where even something as common as a fever could be a sign of further complications and would have to be dealt with immediately or would lead to hospitalization. The hospital had asked my parents to call nightly to notify them of any changes in my health or behaviour.

When I got home from my first biopsy, my dad dropped me off and went out in the rain to buy me a video game on my wish list. It was called "Harvest Moon" and I had fallen in love with it when I had played it at my good friend Matthew's home in Brampton. Whenever I was home between chemo sessions, I would play this game, only stopping to watch "The Price is Right." As my game character grew, I amassed a great fortune, family, multitudes of crops and livestock. My parents would pass by my room and get depressed listening to the sound coming from the game. They hoped that one day I would be able to fulfill in my own life the life I achieved in the game.

On April 19th, I required a surgical procedure at SickKids Hospital to install a port-a-cath in my chest. A port-a-cath, commonly referred to as a port, is a device used to draw blood and give treatments. It is placed under the skin and is attached to a type of central line or catheter. This way the tiny veins in my nine-year-old hands and arms wouldn't get abused. An incision was made on my upper right chest approximately three inches above my nipple. The port was the size of a small hockey puck and protruded with about the same amount of thickness. Prior to my surgery to install the port, the surgeon stressed, "I know you are a very active young man, but please try to be careful not to hit it excessively, like with a bat." This line really stuck with me as, like all kids, I was always playing around, falling, and getting hurt. Every time I fell at school, I would immediately look down my shirt to make sure that my port was still there. After this surgery, I enjoyed eating many freezies in the common area recovery room. For about a week afterward, my chest and arm were sore trying to adjust to this new piece of equipment. It was also not a pleasant time when I had the task of removing the blood-soaked bandages atop the row of stitches on my chest. While bathing, my dad assisted me in removing them as I cringed with every pull.

With the next hockey season approaching and in the midst of my protocol, we decided I would take a sabbatical from hockey. One day I was feeling well, though, so my dad took me to Dave and Busters. Dave and Busters is like a casino for kids with games as far as the eye can see which produce tickets that you can later redeem for a prize. It was there that we ran into my former hockey coach, Neil McNeill, who suggested that I try out for the Vaughan Rangers in the select league. His reasoning was that the select league played half as many games as my former AA league, and was two levels lower. It sounded like a good idea, but first I had to get clearance from my doctor and visit Paul Valenti, our family lawyer, to sign a waiver allowing me to play and accepting any risk that came with it.

Once that was taken care of, my dad and I headed for the first tryout. I was able to stop every puck with ease. Better yet, I completed the goalie races in half the time as it took the other goalies. In the dressing room after the tryout, when I removed my toque while getting undressed, all the other kids and their parents had stunned looks on their faces when they saw my freshly bald head. After the tryout we discussed my situation with the coaching staff and explained that we just didn't know how often I would be able to make it out due to my health and treatment. The coaching staff was so impressed that they were fine with me attending whenever I felt up to it. Very excited to play again, I performed even better at the second tryout.

One week we commuted to SickKids every day for blood tests. By this time, we had a routine in place. It began with me and my dad waking up early to beat the traffic. I often slept in my parents' bedroom at this time since we were leaving together. We would stop at McDonalds for a hotcakes breakfast combo, and then go on to my dad's office at City National Leasing, my pancakes leaving an irresistible trail of a scent behind me until I sat down at his desk to inhale them. Dad's co-workers would all stop in to say hello and ask how I was doing. After my dad completed his work, we would then head off to SickKids Hospital.

We would always use the underground parking at the hospital, usually having to go down to the third or fourth and final level to find a parking spot. As two car enthusiasts, we would point out some of the nicest vehicles while searching for an empty spot and say to one another, "That must belong to a doctor." After parking, we would play another game. Dad would press the upward arrow calling the elevator, while I simultaneously ran into the staircase and up the stairs in an attempt to beat the elevator in a race. I would sprint up the eight to ten flights to either find him waiting at the top or still on his way up. It was a true "boy versus machine" race!

We would then make our way to the 8th floor to register. Along one side of the wall there was usually a lineup, so if we weren't first in line, we would have to wait our turn. Once registered we would wait off to the side to enter a small room to receive a "finger poke." It was always the same nurse who performed the finger pokes. She was a very nice good-hearted woman. I can't recall her name but could sketch her face if I had to. Just before she was ready to poke, she would say, "Okay, ready, 1-2-3 poke!" Once my vial was filled, she would place a sticker with all my information on it and send it wherever it had to go to be tested.

We would then have to wait to be called. Since I'm not a big fan of heights, at first, I wouldn't go near the benches in the hallway as they were extended over air without support. Slowly I came around and began sitting on them and then eventually became very comfortable on them, but I wouldn't look down. While sitting there, my dad and I would often play a game of "I Spy" to pass the time. Alternatively, I would head to the Teen Lounge which was just down the hall. This was a small room for teenagers, but no one seemed to mind that I was only nine years old. In the Teen Lounge was a large big screen television, chairs and board games, a "foosball table" and a video game console which contained my soon-to-be favourite game. It was a baseball game that my dad and I would play all the time while waiting for my name to be called on the overhead speaker system.

Once called, I would report to the oval desk to meet my nurse. Dr. Malkin's nurse was named Mary Stewart. She was a very nice, tall woman whom my family and I got along with well. She would check my height and weight on the other side of the oval desk. I always wanted to be tall, so I was very proud with every millimetre I grew and every pound I put on. Afterwards, I would be called into the blood lab to either have my blood withdrawn and tested or for the purpose of having an intravenous installed. We also got the opportunity to meet several nice nurses in the blood lab over the years. One nurse was actually a friend of my teacher at the time.

The next step was to either head to an arranged appointment or wait for my doctor in a private room, very similar to the one I would stay in for my overnight chemotherapy sessions. In this room, my dad and I often passed time waiting for Dr. Malkin by playing a few games of cards while listening for his footsteps. He would always arrive with his entourage—colleagues and medical students who were shadowing him. He would then call me up to the table to give me a quick physical checkup which often entailed testing my range of vision. He would tell me to follow his pen while he moved it in different directions. Afterwards, he would provide us with any results, announce my protocol for the day and answer any of my parents' questions.

One day, I had strep throat and a fever, with my next chemotherapy session beginning in only a few days. But despite being under the weather, I was excited as I had been invited as a guest of the hospital to watch the Toronto Maple Leafs play the New Jersey Devils in Curtis Joseph's private box. Curtis Joseph's box was located high in the Air Canada Centre. He had donated it for the purposes of lifting the spirits of patients from SickKids. My dad and I and several other children and their families enjoyed our night out, especially the finger foods that were available. Curtis Joseph usually came up to visit his guests in the box after each game, but apparently he lost so much fluid during that game that he had to be connected to an intravenous too. I signed his guestbook and took the memory home with me that night.

On May 4th, we were back at it again, with my second round of chemotherapy. This time my body appeared to be reacting much better to the medicine as I wasn't vomiting nearly as much as the previous time. Once the medicine was complete, I felt good enough to leave my room and roam the halls. I visited the Starlight Lounge for my first and only visit. Then my brother, Justin, arrived and we walked to Marnie's Lounge. Right outside Marnie's Lounge, the wall was painted with all kinds of fun animals which we thought was cool. We really enjoyed this lounge and spent our time playing pool and videogames. As always, I was very competitive, but I had no choice—I was in the fight of my life. That Sunday, I had my first visitor: a teammate of mine, Anthony, and his dad, Clark. They came and brought me an autographed jersey from one of the Maple Leafs players, which I cherished. But over the course of my stay at the hospital, I had very few visitors. In fact, I could probably count them all on one hand. It wasn't because people didn't support me, but because they didn't want to see me in the condition I was in while going through treatment. When I returned home after each session, my grandparents, aunts, uncles, and friends would drop by the house.

During my second session of chemotherapy, a teacher came into my room to speak about the possibility of being "hospital-schooled." She wheeled in with her an interactive learning program on a computer. This game contained cartoon creatures in a forest which tested your mathematical skills. It was very fun and, if I did have to continue learning at the hospital, I was open to it. Fortunately, when I returned home, I felt good enough that I was able to return to grade four at St. Margaret Mary School. Most days, I would arrive about an hour late, as three times each week I had to undergo blood tests at our local clinic. We went there so often that the nurses became very good friends. A nurse by the name of Theresa would draw blood from me most of the time. Since my veins were very small, on a few occasions the nurse had to make two or even three attempts before finding a good blood-drawing vein. I think I was the best customer at the blood clinic during that time period. The nurses there still remember me and ask how I'm doing whenever they bump into my mom.

Afterwards I would get dropped off at school, check in at the office, then walk outside to the portable where my classroom was located. For the first few days of school after a chemotherapy session, I was still not able to eat what my peers were able to. Like Kramer on my favourite show, "Seinfeld," my lunch box would contain one sleeve of soda crackers.

Since my immune system wasn't at par, my mom would ask the teacher to notify us when there was a child with a bad cold or flu in my class so that I could stay home. My two favourite things about school were gym class and recess where I did not hold back due to my illness. During recess, I would play soccer on the field with the older kids, play basketball or play a football game with the boys in my grade as the quarterback for my team. We often had very tough battles that I enjoyed every minute of, because it was better than being on the inside of a hospital.

I got in trouble for my behaviour twice in this period: once for accidentally name-calling someone and another for assisting in pushing a girl in the snow. After the latter, I was sent down to the principal's office with a few others. While pondering what I had just done, I began to think to myself about how I should change my ways. Most of those in the school were aware and sympathetic towards my illness, yet here I was getting into trouble again. As I look back on this now, I wonder whether it was a way of dealing with my feelings about my illness. I did begin to correct my ways during my limited days at school.

On May 14th, we returned to have a follow-up CT scan in order to see how the tumour was reacting to the chemo. A few days later, Dr. Malkin called with great news: there were signs that the tumour was shrinking. I celebrated by making my school's track and field team and playing roller hockey outside with my friends in the neighbourhood. After the first chemo session, my parents had hesitated to send me out to play with my friends. But when I saw my brother going out, I asked, "But why can't I go if Justin gets to go?" My parents reconsidered their decision, feeling that I should have every opportunity that a healthy child has.

My protocol consisted of two methods of delivery for chemotherapy, alternating after every two sessions. After back-to-back in-patient rounds, on May 22nd, I was admitted for my first out-patient round. This meant that I had to travel down every morning from Monday to Friday, staying for twelve hours each day. I was to receive three new chemotherapy medicines, vincristine, dactinomycin and cyclophosphamide. (Try saying that fast!) I would arrive at 7:45 a.m., run up the stairs, register, receive a needle for my intravenous connection, and be ready to begin chemo by 8:30 a.m. The out-patient chemo was administered in the

8th floor's Day Care room which was a few doors away from the Teen Lounge. I remember the Day Care as an all-white room with about ten hospital beds along the walls and three nurses on staff. One of the nurses, Josie, was a friend of my family. I was offered a bed for the day, but without hesitation, I turned it down, wanting to maintain my mobility. Unfortunately, my mobility was limited to the 8th floor alone due to the possibility of an accident occurring. In fact, my chemo medicine was so toxic that if it were to accidentally spill on the floor, the hospital would have to call the fire department to clean it up.

It was a long and gruesome first week as an out-patient, but I soon found out the worst part of it all: the bathroom. In the Day Care there was one designated bathroom for the patients to use. What made going to the bathroom a horror was that every patient had to urinate in their own personal container, all of which would be left on the floor for hours for testing. Just imagine walking into a very small bathroom, and smelling ten people's decomposing urine on the floor. Better yet, we were told to drink as much as possible in order to flush the chemo out of our system by the end of the day. Towards the end of the week, I thought I had found a solution: to wear a mask and hold my breath, but that didn't stand a chance against the urine "kryptonite." My sense of smell also became very annoyed by various scents in the food court. I remember covering my nose with my sleeve as I entered the atrium as the clash of sushi, pasta, soup and more scents would drive me crazy. Reaching the 8th floor was my safe haven during this time period.

That weekend, the annual SickKids telethon was on, I decided to call in to make a personal donation, and then got excited when my name appeared along the bottom of our television. Each year's telethon features various children battling life-threatening illnesses along with their families. One family's story in particular really hit home with my family and me. It was the story of the Matheson family who had two male children battling cancer simultaneously. In fact, one of the children, Spencer Matheson, shared both my type of cancer and my oncologist, Dr. David Malkin. In Spencer's case, his tumour kept returning rapidly, leaving the doctors no other option but to remove the tumour along with his eye. Watching this first telethon after my diagnosis inspired my family to start thinking of ways that we, too, could give back to this great hospital.

On June 11th, I was back at it again for my fourth round of chemo. Yet again I decided to forego the hospital bed I was offered in the Day Care room. I spent most of my time in one of the game rooms or at the far end of the 8th floor where there were several wooden benches. This was a nice and quiet area, much less travelled than the wing closest to the clinic. The benches were in front of a wall of windows, the only place where it was possible to see out into the world. It was even possible to soak up some rays on a sunny day.

But this round of chemo was a little tougher. My dad recalls that after I vomited for the fourth or fifth time in one day, I lifted my head from the pail and said, "I feel like having a hot dog, but I don't think I should." I must have caught a glimpse of the hot dog vendor stationed outside the entrance to the hospital. That day I didn't have a hot dog, but a few times throughout my treatment my dad and I wheeled out to grab one when I felt well enough.

At the conclusion of the week, Dr. Malkin scheduled a CT scan before my next chemotherapy session. Based on the results of the scan, he would then decide whether I required radiation therapy or surgery. If by chance the cancer was gone, then we would just continue with chemo.

Before I left the hospital, we decided to follow through on our plans to give back to SickKids by visiting the SickKids Foundation office to talk about how we could start fundraising for the hospital.

On June 21st, my dad and I drove downtown to our consultation with my soon-to-be radiologist from Princess Margaret Hospital, Dr. Laperriere. Prior to doing so, I passed by SickKids to drop off a big box of books donated courtesy of Penguin Books through a customer of my father.

"Andrew's radiation protocol would include receiving radiation therapy every day for five consecutive weeks," said Dr. Laperriere, going on to explain how radiation affects the cancer cells, stopping them from growing. As with anything, there were harmful side effects which included the following: the rays that passed through my head might in time cause non-related tumour growth in other areas; in two years, I would probably develop a cataract in my left eye; I might have some vision damage in my left eye; that portion of my face and eye area might not grow to its normal capacity; my growth hormones might also be affected. Dr. Laperriere concluded by saying, "Most of these side effects could be corrected with surgery or drugs." Looking back, it appears that the cons were plenty, but at the time, my only comment was: "I hope it doesn't affect my height, because I need to be tall in order to be a good basketball player."

Four days later on June 25th, I got sized for a new mask. This time it wasn't for a goalie mask, but a radiation mask that would be used to protect the rest of my face from the radiation's harmful rays. I had to lay still in a small office in Princess Margaret Hospital, while a doctor began by wrapping my head with saran wrap, followed by a plaster-like substance. Once hardened, it became a perfect mould of my face. From this a clear mask was made which, for me, resembled the mask worn in the movie *Hollow Man*. On our way out of the hospital, my dad and I purchased a ticket for the Princess Margaret Lottery in the lobby. Then I ended the day back at SickKids for another CT scan and a finger poke.

That night, Dr. Malkin called with the results of the CT scan. It seemed that there was a relationship between quick calls and bad news. In fact, that again was the case. Dr. Malkin said, "The swelling on the top of Andrew's eye could be a benign muscle growth or a benign tumour that is not reacting to the chemo. If that is the case, then different cancer-fighting medicines could be used." He continued, "If it is benign, then the continuation of chemotherapy would shrink it over time." Before the radiation began, my medical staff wanted to see what exactly they were dealing with. Hence, another biopsy was scheduled with my good surgeon, Dr. Pashby.

Towards the end of June another CT scan was scheduled, at Princess Margaret Hospital this time. Following the scan, I got to test out my new radiation mask which my dad said made me look like a mannequin. On July 10th my biopsy was conducted. By this time, I was a veteran and knew exactly what to expect. After a successful biopsy and a quick recovery, Dr. Malkin called two days later with the good news we were all praying for. The tissue tested from the biopsy contained no signs of cancer.

FOUR
Radioactive Boy

I wasn't thrilled that Monday July 16 would be the first of my upcoming twenty-five radiation sessions, as my family had rented a condo in Collingwood for the last two weeks of July. Collingwood is located about an hour and a half northwest of where we live, and my family has a tradition of renting there every summer. It's a beautiful community, impeccably maintained and filled with the friendliest of people. I always found it nice there when complete strangers waved and said hi to us. We would enjoy such activities as swimming, tennis, barbequing, watching movies, playing family board games and more.

But I didn't have a choice. With my mother and brothers up north, my dad and I got up early to beat the always-congested traffic into the city. Since SickKids didn't have the capability to perform radiation, my therapy was held across the street at Princess Margaret Hospital. The radiation wing is located on the lower level of the hospital. As I walked down the stairs for the first time and every time afterwards, I would be the target of lots of stares. Since most people there were more than five times my age, they rarely witnessed someone as young as me walk in. While my mature neighbours in the radiation wing were often preoccupied with reading magazines, I would take advantage of the sole computer in the corner which was intended for important patient use. I quickly realized that it contained the game "Space Pinball," and I figured, what could be more important than pinball? Needless to say, during the next five weeks I became a pro at pinball.

Once my name was called, I entered into a hallway that contained a huge vault-like metal door behind which the radiation therapy took place. Radiation therapy uses high energy radiation to kill cancer cells. Pioneered in late 1899 by German physics professor, Wilhelm Conrad Roentgen, it works by damaging cells over and over. It can also damage normal cells along with cancer cells, therefore treatment has to be carefully planned to minimize side effects.

My first session was the longest of them all. First we had to meet the technicians who would be assisting me throughout my treatments. They were two very nice ladies. One of them was British and took the time to teach me a word every day, two of which I remember—"loo" which means bathroom and "lorry" which means a truck—although I often got these two words confused with one another. Before we began, a few adjustments had to be made to my mask to secure a proper fit. Once everything was sorted out, I was told to lie very still on the bed which had an overhanging element above my head that provided the radiation. The actual treatment took between ten and fifteen minutes to complete and didn't affect the way I felt at all. I just hoped that the radiation was frying my cancer cells. On my second day of radiation, I made a discovery of Columbus-discovering-America proportions. There was a huge playroom available to radiation patients which had such items as a basketball game like something you'd see at a carnival, a large green jungle gym, and a big screen television with a gaming console. This fun room combined with the computer's Space Pinball made the journey more enjoyable.

The rest of my first week of radiation flew by and then my dad and I joined the rest of my family in Collingwood. Knowing what I had to look forward to come Monday, this weekend I had a blast. I got to experience my first ride in a beautiful Corvette, my first time driving a boat, and going tubing, and capped it off with getting a basketball net which I had long asked for. In fact, my parents bought me the basketball net only because I promised to attend Camp Oochigeas the following summer.

Camp Oochigeas is a privately funded summer camp and program offered by SickKids for patients battling cancer and other diseases. "Camp Ooch" as it's known is actually the only residential camp in the province of Ontario to offer IV chemotherapy and blood transfusions on-site, so even children in the intense phase of their cancer treatment can still experience camp. I held back for a while since I had never gone to camp before and wouldn't know anybody, but I finally gave in. Unfortunately, I never got a chance to fulfill my end of the promise.

I breezed through the remaining four weeks of radiation. Towards the end, my family noticed a soft bald spot had formed on the back of my head directly behind the eye area. I thought to myself, *wow, that's one strong laser*! For my very last session, my mother and brothers came to join me for added support. As the radiation machine shut off for the final time, I felt an overwhelming sense of pride and accomplishment having completed my radiation. I walked out of that vault door with my head held high and said farewell to the fabulous nurses who had treated me for the last five weeks. The cherry on top was that I got to take home my radiation mask, a toy bear I named Tiger which had kept me company throughout my treatments, along with my calendar of stickers commemorating each session.

To celebrate, my family all went to the CN Tower's revolving restaurant for lunch. It was a long ride up and, as the elevator doors opened, I couldn't hear a thing as my ears popped. My family knows I'm not the biggest fan of heights, so I made sure I took the farthest seat from the window. The view from the top was spectacular! I remember saying, "Dad, we could probably see our house from here." The food, though, was a little too fancy for my taste. I ordered some kind of meat with mashed potatoes. I don't recall how the meat was, but the bed of mashed potatoes was delicious. Having just overcome five weeks of radiation made them taste even better.

That same night I had a hockey practice at six. While at the rink, I found out that my brother's team, which was playing across the hall at seven, was short a goalie. So after finishing my practice, I headed to yet another. My dad suggested, "Maybe all that radiation has given you super powers." I glanced back and smiled.

FIVE
Chemo Round #2

I was very excited to be starting grade five. I woke up at 6:30 a.m. on the first day of school, excited in anticipation of this new beginning. There were two grade five teachers at the time with two very opposite reputations. Due to my situation, the school and my parents thought it would be a good idea to place me with the teacher with the good reputation. But as the nice teacher called out the list of names the students in her class, I got ready to step forward with every name called, but istead I was called into the so-called "mean" teacher's class. I carried on and got set up in my new classroom. A few hours later I was called to the office and was told that a mistake had been made and that I was supposed to be placed in the other classroom. I was given the option of changing if I desired, but for whatever reason, I decided to stay put.

Looking back, I made the right decision and I carry that trait with me today. When I'm at a restaurant and I receive the wrong order, as long as it's within reason, I will accept my fate and move forward. (My mother, on the other hand, will always order the most specific item on the menu and it always shows up at our table wrong. She has no problem sending it back to the kitchen. It drives me crazy sometimes, so I tell her to "Just eat it already." She responds, "No, I ordered what I ordered and expect to receive it!")

I treated cancer with that same attitude. I was handpicked out of thousands, so all I could do is choose to accept it, fight, and press on. There's no sense feeling sorry for yourself or seeking sympathy from others.

On the medical side, it was my first week in six months free of any blood tests or needles. It was also over two months since my last round of chemo, and I had a tremendous increase in energy. Even my hair had started to grow back. I had had my dad time me while I ran laps around our court while it was pitch black outside.

But my stint of being needle-free was rather short-lived, as I was scheduled for an assessment at SickKids next week, followed by a minor surgical procedure two days later. It seems that my eye wasn't healing correctly after the latest biopsy so Dr. Pashby would be draining the fluid under my eye with the goal of reducing the swelling. The surgery was yet again a success. Afterwards, Dr. Pashby, in a conversation with my dad, said, "If Andrew had been diagnosed twenty years ago with the same cancer, he would have had no chance."

In the meantime, we had moved ahead with our plans to raise money with a fundraising banquet on October 12 for SickKids. Because my parents didn't have fundraising experience and didn't know where to start, the owner of the banquet hall suggested we talk to someone named Sam Ciccolini. Sam is a successful businessman originally from our region of Italy. He is also a well-known philanthropist who was on the board of SickKids for ten years and received the Order of Canada for his good work. He also lost his daughter Cristina when she was ten. He gave good advice to my dad about how to raise money for SickKids. We received an array of support for our banquet, including corporate donations and gifts, media coverage, and celebrities interested in attending. Within minutes of the first media profile about our fundraiser, we received a flurry of calls from local supporters. The phone rang one night and my dad answered it. It was a woman named Nancy who had seen the article in the paper and wanted to share her son David's story. It turned out that fifteen years before, David had been diagnosed with the same type of cancer, in the same location, at the same age as me. My dad started to get goosebumps while hearing such an unexpected and comforting story. David was now twenty-four years old, had just become an architect, and was getting married next year. This story gave my family some much-needed hope.

A few days later I was back at SickKids. Just prior to my next round of chemo, we received the results from my assessment. Dr. Malkin explained, "You're doing well, and will hopefully only need four more treatments of chemotherapy." He continued, "Next month you'll have to have a CT scan to determine the results of the radiation treatment you received." Before the conversation ended, my parents picked his brain regarding the amazing research he was doing in his lab, specifically regarding the encouraging results he was getting with vitamin A on rhabdo tumors. He explained: "When vitamin A is introduced, the cancer cells turn into muscle tissue." He continued: "I hope that one day a child diagnosed with Andrew's disease will not require chemotherapy or radiation." This inspired us to raise as much money as possible at our upcoming fundraiser.

Shortly after, I was admitted for my second round of chemotherapy, post-radiation. This time it was conducted as an in-patient over a three-day period. As it was in the beginning, so it was again, me with my nausea, watching "The Price is Right," and my dad finding it difficult to sleep on the uncomfortable bedside couch. By this time, I had played my Sega baseball game so often that I was no longer amused by it.

Since we always carried my yellow and blue hospital backpack around wherever we went, it made it easy for us to verify whether what I was receiving was accurate or not. Luckily for me, in a few instances, my dad caught a nurse accidentally attempting to give me the wrong medicine.

On October 1st, I was back for chemotherapy as an out-patient. That meant five twelve-hour days lay ahead. This time, the mixture of medicines made me more nauseated than in the past. One day I actually elected to reserve a hospital bed and lie down for the day. We chose the bed in the farthest and quietest corner. I had just finished vomiting several times, felt very weak and was thirsty. My dad went down to get me a drink and came back with blue Powerade. I drank about half the bottle before I began to feel nauseated again. My poor dad had the task of mopping up the sticky blue liquid from the floor and a few drops that landed on my bed. As for me, even today, when given the choice between types of Powerade, I'll never choose blue.

In the bed adjacent to me was another father and son who witnessed the whole incident. I don't recall too much, given my state at the time, but the son was a few years my junior and the father worked as a miner. I thought that was a very interesting occupation, as I had never met a miner before. Like many at SickKids, they had travelled from another province of Canada to receive the best treatment available in the country. They were staying at The Ronald McDonald House which provides a home for out-of-town families with sick children.

During my stay at SickKids, we developed a close bond with several other families as we shared in the same struggle. We came to know Brandon Desousa and his family. Brandon was battling leukemia and was undergoing blood transfusions in the Day Care room frequently. My mother and his mother would often chat. There was also Michael and his father, whom we would see all the time. Often, children would wear a piece of clothing to distinguish them or perhaps motivate them during the struggle. Michael would always wear a Maple Leafs jersey and was around the same age as me. There was also a female teenager who my Mom called "Kappa Girl," since she was always wearing the brand Kappa's tracksuits. There were several other families and patients we got to know, but these ones were the most memorable.

One day after school, I entered through the front door of my house, threw my bag on the floor and headed straight to the kitchen for a snack as always. On my way up the stairs, my dad called me into his bedroom in a soft voice. He said, "Andrew, sit down for a minute." I sat on his bed as he continued, "You know Brandon was also very sick, right?" I nodded. He continued, "Well, he passed away yesterday." I didn't know what to say, so I left the room shortly after. My parents visited the funeral home to see Brandon one last time. This wasn't the last time I would be called into my parents' room after school to be given such sad news. I don't know what ended up happening to the miner's son, Michael, or to Kappa girl, but I hope that they are able to read these very words.

After this past round of chemo, my hair had begun to fall out again. Instead of allowing my hair to shed all over the house, my dad decided to bribe me to shave my head again. This time, for whatever reason, a lacrosse racket was on my mind. Now, I had never played organized lacrosse, but thought it was a cool sport. So I gave into the bribe, but I didn't let him cut my hair before I pulled a trick on my friends at school. One day when I went to the bathroom at school, I touched my hair to style it as I looked in the mirror. As I lowered my hand, I noticed that I had accidentally pulled out a chunk of my hair. I quickly called a few friends of mine to join me in the bathroom as I said, "Watch this!" I then easily pulled out a big chunk of my hair, astonishing my friends.

The following week I was busy promoting our upcoming fundraiser. On Saturday I attended my first-ever golf tournament, while on Sunday, I was on television for the first time. The producer of the show said, "I want to tell Andrew's story, and how he has been an inspiration battling his cancer." The story would air on the next SickKids telethon.

October 12th finally arrived and four hundred people were on hand for the Andrew Mizzoni Charity Dinner Dance Gala. A few months prior I had been the ring bearer for my cousin's wedding and had gotten to wear a very nice tuxedo. So when faced with the question of what to wear to the dinner dance, I thought a tuxedo was the way to go. I wore my beautiful black tux, combined with a silver tie, vest, and cufflinks to complete the attire. For days leading up to the event, my dad mentioned that I was going to get a ride from someone special. At the time, I didn't have a clue what this meant. So in my regular fashion, I asked a million questions, "By who? A man? Woman? Do I know them? What's their name? Why?" All I was able to get out of my dad was that it was a woman named Vivian Black. Suspense built up in me as the event drew near.

On the night of the event, the doorbell rang. I ran down the stairs as I always did to open the door. To my surprise, on the other side of the door was a blonde woman who said, "You must be Andrew. I am a friend of your dad's and I am going to be your ride to the banquet hall." Still not sure why she was giving me a ride, I took one step out the door and saw a beautiful black BMW Z3 roadster convertible in my driveway. It was just like the one Pierce Brosnan drove as James Bond. It turned out that Vivian worked for BMW of Mississauga, and my dad had done business with her in the past. When my dad mentioned the event we were having, she graciously offered to provide me a ride. Before we left the house, she handed me a bag full of BMW merchandise such as a Ralf Schumacher F1 model car, a wind-up BMW toy car, a key chain, a book, and a hat, among other things.

I then posed for a picture standing in front of the car in my driveway. There I was, rain falling, black car, black tuxedo, bald head, as the camera snapped. To this day, I keep that picture next to my bed for daily inspiration.

On the ride to the banquet hall, Vivian drove well and fast. She told me, "I drove the BMW F1 racing car around a track several times, the same car that Ralf Schumacher drives." I thought that was very cool as Ralf Schumacher was one of the biggest names in racing at the time, and brother of Ferrari's Michael Schumacher. Too bad the hall was only five minutes away from our home, because I would have loved to experience the car perform for longer.

As I entered the hall I was amazed at how great everything looked. Just outside the main hall was a table with my hockey jersey, gear and even my radiation mask which guests stopped to see upon entering. Inside the hall were over forty tables filled with family, friends, teammates, medical staff, politicians, and celebrities. During dinner, I sat next to one of the greatest goaltenders of all time, Johnny Bower, and his lovely wife. He shared many stories including one about how his teammate Eddy Shack stole his Stanley Cup Championship ring. We then both autographed the bottom of a dinner plate, which I still have to this day. At the end of the night, I gave a speech, in which I mentioned our plans of having a charity golf tournament the following summer. After a long day and after having such a good time, I fell asleep on the couch in the lobby of the banquet hall. I later heard that everyone said goodbye to me as they exited the hall. We ended up raising $40,000 that night to support pediatric cancer research at SickKids Hospital.

Two days later, it was Thanksgiving weekend and my tenth birthday. It's amazing how drastically life could change in only a year's time. I enjoyed my tenth birthday fully and took nothing for granted. The following week, leading up to another round of chemotherapy, was filled with tremendous experiences at Toronto sporting events. First, my dad, my brother Justin, and I were guests of Michael "Pinball" Clemons, the coach at the time and a former star of the CFL's Toronto Argonauts football team. After hearing about my battle with cancer, Pinball volunteered to support my fundraiser and family in any way he could. Pinball is an amazing, well-respected man in Toronto and the national football community, and has a smile that could light up a room. We were able to watch the game from the field, standing right next to players who were three times the size of me. It was a great game. Afterwards we were lucky enough to go in the locker room to meet all the players. My brother and I got every player on the team to autograph the back of our Argo jerseys. But for me the highlight of the game was when I was photographed surrounded by about ten gorgeous cheerleaders! Could you believe I was afraid at first to be in the picture? What a mistake that would have been!

Next on the agenda were two platinum tickets to see the Toronto Raptors basketball team take on Michael Jordan's Washington Wizards courtesy of my Uncle Danny. It, too, was an amazing game with high flying plays performed by none other than Vince Carter. After the game, we ran into some family friends of ours and a teammate on my hockey team. We told them that we were looking for Pinball who had earlier told my dad that he, too, was going to the game. Our friends pointed us in Pinball's direction which was literally two rows from where we were sitting. Pinball asked if we had some time available, having already known that I was scheduled for chemo at eleven that same night. He then took me and my dad down to the court, through the tunnel, to just outside the Raptors dressing room. One by one, I got the opportunity to meet the players as they exited the dressing room.

Then Pinball introduced us to Vince Carter's mom, Michelle. She was a lovely lady. My dad and Michelle spoke about their respective children. I remember her saying, "My son is always the last to leave the dressing room, because he likes to look his best." She then took us into a small room just inside the dressing room doors used for post-game interviews. A few minutes later, in walked Vince Carter wearing a black dress shirt and gray pants. I was in awe as my dad told Vince about our fundraiser. Vince asked me, "Did you enjoy the game?" I must have smiled ear to ear as the Raptors were victorious and Vince was the star with thirty-one points over Michael's twenty-two. Vince signed the front of my jersey and my dad snapped a photo of me and Vince. That photo was later published in several publications, in which one was titled, "Heroes Big and Small." It was an amazing experience but it wasn't over yet, as on our way out I heard a lot of commotion. As I glanced over my left shoulder I saw one of the best athletes ever, Michael Jordan. He was about ten feet away from me as he walked by surrounded by a crowd of people.

We thanked Pinball for the experience and then took the short drive from the Air Canada Centre to SickKids. I remember walking up to the in-patient registration desk and telling all the nurses about the night we just had. Once my room was ready, I carefully took off the jersey, folded it and placed it in one of the drawers under the couch where my dad would sleep.

I got hooked up and ready for another round of chemotherapy. This time I was very ill and couldn't eat or drink anything. Time also felt as if it was standing still, as I watched the clock across my bed tick all day. I had even brought a little basketball net and hung it on the bathroom door but I was too weak to play. I was scheduled to go down to the foundation to present them with the funds raised from our fundraiser, but I couldn't make the trip. The presentation was instead made in my room while I slept, with the understanding that we would take the celebratory photo on my next visit. After three very long days of this, I finally got to go home. Fortunately, I quickly bounced back and began eating as soon as I got home.

A few days later I brought home my school portrait for grade five. I was disappointed with the way it turned out. My parents asked, "Is it because of your hair?" I replied, "No." They continued, "Is it because you've lost your eyebrows?" I said, "No" again. Then they asked, "Well then, what is it?" I answered, "I don't like how I smiled." As a ten-year-old, I was oblivious to what others thought about my hair and cared only about my crooked smile.

Before I knew it, I was back at SickKids for what my protocol called my final round of chemotherapy. This time it went a lot smoother than the last time but had the reverse effect as I was sick only after leaving the hospital. To make matters more complicated, I had to perform my first radio interview over the phone in support of the SickKids Radio-thon with Mix 99.9, a popular Toronto radio station. Given the circumstances, I think I did quite well, accompanied by my vomit bowl the entire time.

On December 4, I was scheduled to return to SickKids for some tests to determine if I was going to continue with more chemotherapy or graduate to a three-month follow-up stage. After the testing, we met with Dr. Malkin who said, "In ten years I have only had six cases of kids with the same cancer as Andrew's, and only one child's cancer returned." The odds seemed favourable, and we waited and prayed for good news. We soon received a call which would determine which statistic I was going to fall under.

SIX
Remission

Some cancer patients will admit that the toughest part of treatment is not the treatment itself, but the time after the treatment: remission. This was the case for me as some of my very lowest points came after my cancer was done, and they might have even seemed unrelated to cancer. It was also true for someone who was, and still remains, a symbol of hope for the cancer community: cyclist Lance Armstrong. Lance found it very difficult during remission, as he attended monthly checkups with a sense of dread that he might hear the words, "You have cancer" uttered again. With every passing month and after many nights of stress and anxiety, the chances of a relapse lessened and Lance continued doing what he loved to do, with much success. I've always found him to be inspirational and I often wear my Livestrong shoes, tracksuit and wristband. When I do, people often tell me, "You know he cheated, right?" as if I've been in a cave all my life. I did feel a little betrayed when he finally confessed to steroid use after so many denials, but even if he is stripped of his Tour De France titles and his reputation, it doesn't change the fight he won with cancer.

It was December 6, 2001, when my oncologist called with the news that my cancer was now in remission. My family's prayers had been answered. For three full months I would not have to see the inside of a hospital or feel another prick of a needle. This was such a relief for me, and for the first time in ten months, I could get back to being a normal ten-year-old boy again. I quickly began playing hockey with a surge of new energy. Before I knew it, my hair began to grow back –and it wasn't curly! My parents received an unexpected call from the Children's Wish Foundation with some more great news. They would be granting my wish and sending my entire family to Florida's Walt Disney World, in March. I was thrilled!

Ironically, I ended 2001 back in the hospital after my brother Justin tackled me while playing football on New Year's Eve, and I cracked my head on a table—but that was nothing four stitches couldn't repair.

I underwent some bloodwork and another CT scan on February 25, 2002. A few days later Dr. Malkin called with the good news that my results showed no sign of cancer. In three months I was scheduled for my second round of post-cancer testing. If those results were also positive, we would proceed to remove my port-a-cath which was still inside my upper right chest. Unlike Lance, I never really got stressed-out thinking if my cancer would return. But, then again, I was a quiet ten-year-old kid.

March quickly arrived and my family and I boarded a plane to visit every kid's dream, Disney World, courtesy of the Children's Wish Foundation. For those unfamiliar with it, the Children's Wish Foundation helps grant wishes of children battling life-threatening illnesses. The Children's Wish Foundation generously took care of all the expenses of the resort, family passes to all the theme parks, a rental vehicle, and even spending money. We used a portion of the spending money to purchase a video camera to capture these special moments. We had an amazing time at the resort, the different theme parks, and eating at several buffets. We enjoyed many hours of great moments, caught on the video camera, which we'll cherish for years. I had had lots of medicine over the last twelve months, but this getaway was the best kind of medicine any child could ask for.

I was scheduled for my next round of testing on May 27. If the results followed the likes of those prior, then I would graduate to a longer follow-up period, have my port removed, and, in essence, put cancer behind me forever.

SEVEN
The Relapse

It was nearly six months since my last round of chemotherapy and my remission was a time of bliss. Planning was well underway for our first golf tournament fundraiser. But the results of my latest tests had arrived and Dr. Malkin had called us into his office to show us the results. When we arrived, Dr. Malkin was gazing at an image on his computer screen. On the screen were my CT scan results which were being compared in a split-screen format with my earlier results. He showed us some fragments which were not visible in my earlier scan but were now present. He said, "It is possible the area of concern is due to the radiation treatment from the summer, but, if it is cancerous, my concern is how quick it's progressing after six months." He decided to schedule an immediate biopsy. Being a biopsy veteran by now, I no longer had any confusion between that word and autopsy. I honestly don't remember any immense sadness after hearing that I might have cancer again, but looking back, I could see how hard it must have been for my parents to accept this news.

Dr. Hurwitz performed my biopsy a few days later. It went successfully without any complications. The samples removed were sent to Dr. Malkin's lab for testing. Two long days passed before my family would hear the words uttered from my doctor's mouth for the second time: "Andrew has cancer." Still, the extent of the cancer was unknown until I underwent a myriad of tests again. Since rhabdomyosarcoma is a fast-growing type of cancer, and given the time the cancer had to spread over the last six months, we were really praying for the best. Four days after finding out my cancer had returned, I was scheduled for what would be my ninth round of chemotherapy. Dr. Malkin and his staff were optimistic that the cancer had not spread, but we wouldn't be sure for a few days.

A few months earlier, my dad had set up a page about my battle on the CaringBridge network. CaringBridge [https://www.caringbridge.org/] is a non-profit service that connects family and friends to share information, love, and support when someone is facing a serious medical condition. On my page, my dad had posted my story, uploading pictures, and documenting my treatments. My site was getting thousands of viewers weekly. I remember when my dad would say, "Guess how many hits you got today?" We made a game out of it, and he said: "When we get to 50,000 viewers, we'll do something special." We surpassed 50,000 viewers and went out for a special family dinner to celebrate. There was also a guestbook portion of the website where people from all over the world, including family and friends, would post inspiring messages. Looking back at the website, I realized that my dad posted "Pray for Andrew" in various ways after several of his posts, especially as we waited to know what the progress of the cancer had been. I don't doubt that those prayers aided in my recovery. "And the prayer of faith shall save the sick, and the Lord shall raise him up" (James 5:15, KJV).

The news prayed for had finally been delivered, and it was good news: the cancer was contained in my orbital region and had not spread to other parts of my body. My protocol consisted of several months of much harsher chemotherapy through different medicines. If these medicines were ineffective, I would require radical surgery. It was also at this time that I was made aware that children could actually tolerate more chemotherapy than adults, possibly because children are less likely to have incurred other health issues such as heart disease, kidney disease, lung disease or diabetes. This news pumped me up as I prepared for a three-day stint of chemotherapy.

I would receive two different medicines, cisplatin and dauxorubicin. Both are used to treat and kill various types of cancer. Interestingly enough, cisplatin is actually a soluble form of platinum, and was the drug used to treat Lance Armstrong's testicular cancer. It does have some nasty side effects though, such as intense nausea and kidney damage. Nerve damage and hearing loss are also common side-effects and were why I would have to have semi-annual hearing and heart tests conducted at SickKids for years afterwards. And this round of chemo did live up to its reputation of making me very ill. My vomit bowl had never seen as much action as it did at that stage, as vomiting was one of the only activities I was capable of performing.

I received some visitors from the United States that week who had heard about me from my CaringBridge site. Unfortunately, I was in no state to offer any type of hospitality when they arrived. From what I remember, it was a mother, two children and their friends. They were very friendly people and I think they even brought me a gift. I was feeling very weak. I had brought my basketball net again which was affixed to the bathroom door in hopes of shooting from my bed but sadly, I think I may have only taken two shots during my entire stay. I was happier than ever to leave the hospital after three long days in hopes of my health improving. Unfortunately, I didn't make it farther than the underground parking garage before I vomited, this time in the backseat of my dad's car. My dad is precise about maintaining a clean car, so luckily for him and his car, I had a vomit bowl with me and my aim had improved greatly over the last two years.

One evening only a few days after leaving the hospital from chemotherapy, I found myself fighting a fever. I lay on our couch with a cold facecloth on my forehead in an attempt to lessen the fever but it didn't go down, so my parents decided that I should go directly to SickKids as they had been told to do if this scenario were to occur. I was in a "neutropenic" state at the time, which meant that my immune system was weak and I was susceptible to viruses. My dad and I took off to SickKids Hospital and checked into Emergency, a place I'd seen but never entered before. Due to the high volume of patients, we waited in the hallway for a long period of time before I was given my own room. I don't remember much as I was feeling woozy and fatigued at the time, but I remember lying in a semi-private room on a bed until I could be transferred to a suitable location. Because the hospital was at full capacity I was stationed in a hospital room outside of the eighth floor Oncology wing. I was kept on watch and given some medication to assist with bringing my fever down. We were told that I had to remain hospitalized until my fever had been gone for more than forty-eight hours.

My cousin Julianna came to visit me unexpectedly on her own and to bring me a gift, a Spider Man game for my PlayStation. Her presence made the world of a difference and is something I'll always remember. For this reason, when I hear someone is in the hospital, I always try my best to visit, because I know it will mean a lot for them as it did for me. The following day, my grandparents, John and Esther Mizzoni, came to visit us. I enjoyed playing a few games of cards to pass the time with my *nonna* who I liked to call Gramps. Towards the end of the day, my grandparents sensed my dad's fatigue and my grandfather offered to stay with me for a few days.

Gramps stayed and our "Go Fish" marathon began. We played for a quarter a game and I put my winnings in an empty purple Gobstoppers candy box. I think I accumulated close to eight dollars by the time he left. My grandfather was a great storyteller, so I would ask questions that fueled him telling his stories about working at the railroad, or about his fictional horses. He also admired beauty, and I recall him whistling at one lady as we passed her in the food court. She looked back to see who the perpetrator was. I hope she didn't think it was me!

That night I experienced excruciating pain in my lower back which kept me from sleeping. The nurses would eventually give me something intravenously to help stop the pain, but in the meantime, Gramps held a cold cloth against the area. I was being monitored every few hours with an automatic thermometer in place under my tongue. As hour forty was approaching, my temperature rose to an unacceptable level, and my stay had to be lengthened by at least another two days. Space was now available on the eighth floor, so I was moved to a comfortable room there.

By the time I was feverless, I had been at the hospital for almost an entire week. It was my longest overnight stay at "Hotel SickKids," and it was because of a side effect of the chemo medication. Afterwards, we were told by my doctor that I had been lucky I had only suffered a fever once. Apparently, it's common that patients experience several fevers, along with blood levels that require them to receive blood transfusions throughout their treatment. So, in the end, I was blessed that it was just this single occurrence.

The first Andrew Mizzoni Charity Golf Classic was approaching and was already sold out. I was also going to have my name recognized on the donor wall at SickKids Hospital, a wall that recognizes individuals whose cumulative contributions have reached or exceeded $25,000, and corporations, foundations, associations and community events that have generously given $50,000 or more, since April 1, 1993. On one of our trips to Kleinburg Golf Course, where the event was held, my dad took my brother and I to his parents' house, which was right around the corner. After playing tennis at our cousin's house next door, I ran inside to quench my thirst. As I poured myself a glass of water I glanced at the calendar on the front of the fridge. I had lost track of the days and couldn't believe that my two weeks of grace was almost up and I was already due back for my next round of chemotherapy.

In no time at all, I was hooked up to my intravenous and being injected with chemo medicine. This time was evidently no better than the last time. Dr. Malkin confided that, "We will wait for three weeks to see the full results of the chemotherapy, and then start planning for the surgery next month." I was accepting whatever route my journey had to go.

Towards the final hours of this round of chemo, my dad and I saw a nurse in the halls carrying a large box. In her box was an assortment of beads which could be used to make a necklace referred to as "bravery beads." There were various colours to choose from, each of which symbolized a particular treatment or procedure. My dad went through the list saying, "Yes, you had one of these, some of these, and we can't forget some of these." I quickly realized that my necklace would be three feet long if I put everything I had undergone on it so I had no choice but to cap it. I did add beads to spell out my name, as well as a basketball, soccer ball bead and a bear that is the hospital's logo. The final knot was tied to complete the necklace and I displayed it proudly on the top of my intravenous during the remainder of my stays at the hospital. Today, I have wrapped my bravery beads around the rearview mirror in my car. Every time someone new enters my car, they can't help but ask about the significance of the beads. A few times I've even been told, "Nice Mardi Gras beads."

There were only a few weeks remaining in the school year when I returned to school after this round of chemotherapy on the very day our regional track and field meet happened to be taking place. Having already made the relay team for my age, I elected to participate at the meet. It was held at a local university and included hundreds of students from grades three to eight. I remember it was a beautiful sunny day and I was wearing my blue Italian soccer jersey, as the World Cup was taking place around this same time. With very little training leading up to the meet, I was the second runner. As my teammate came around the corner of one of the inside lanes, I accepted the baton cleanly and was off on the straight-away. The race was neck and neck throughout the halfway point of my portion when the competitor to my right entered my lane throwing my running motion off in disarray. Unable to regain my balance, I came tumbling down. By the time I was back up on my feet, it was too late: the racers had advanced too far as the official raised his flag to disqualify the other team that led to our downfall. As I walked up to my teammates, I felt very badly that we were not able to win the race. We came in 6th place (although in succeeding years we would come in first!). The teachers on hand for the meet were very worried about my state, despite me saying I was fine several times. They called my mother to notify her of what had taken place. My mom was shocked that I had even attended, having just been released from the hospital only days prior. I was fortunate to drive back to the school with a few teachers, who were nice enough to buy ice cream on the way.

Two weeks later our golf tournament was wildly successful, raising another $22,000 for SickKids Hospital. Everyone on hand had a wonderful time, and even the Toronto Argonaut cheerleaders made an appearance. At this event the Toronto Raptors' mascot was present during registration. I remember him doing all kinds of fun stuff including flips on the tee of the first hole. He even allowed me to hit a ball which he placed on the tip of his nose. I felt a little badly, as along with hitting the ball, I hit a piece of his nose.

One week later, my CT scan results were in. It appeared that although the tumour hadn't grown, at the same time there was no indication of it shrinking either. The bittersweet news caused my doctor to schedule another five-day cycle of chemotherapy as an out-patient. I was prescribed a combination of the drug cyclophosphamide along with a new drug called topotican. My body reacted to this new cocktail of chemo very well. Afterwards, in the evening, I even played basketball and tennis outside of my house. Since I had to return the next day during out-patient chemotherapy, my nurses left a needle and attachment connected to my port for a quicker setup. I remember being cautious not to hit it while playing, as well as showing it off under my shirt to my friends on the street.

The next day I felt great at SickKids, so when the medicine was complete and I was getting flushed, my dad and I left the hospital. IV in hand, we walked out the front doors and down the street to my favourite restaurant, The Devil's Advocate. I wasn't too crazy about the name but I also thought it sounded cool. At that time, there was smoking allowed in restaurants and, since it was a pub, I was only allowed to eat on the patio. That was fine with me after having been inside a hospital all day. I always ordered my favourite meal: fajitas. They came scorching hot on a skillet combined with the sides of cheese, peppers, onions and salsa. For dessert, I ordered another family favourite: apple crumble pie. This place became a little place of serenity away from the hospital until, of course, my IV started beeping as a reminder to return to the hospital to renew my medicine. For sentimental reasons, even today, I make a point of stopping by that restaurant whenever I am in the area. The name of the restaurant has now changed to The Duke of Somerset and the menu no longer offers fajitas and apple crumble, but it will always have a special place in my heart.

That night we received a call from the hospital. This time it wasn't for any test results, but to let us know that my hero, Curtis Joseph, would be holding a meeting the next day at the hospital after my chemo. It happened that Cujo had been traded to the Detroit Red Wings and he was announcing his continued support and funding of the "Cujo's Kids" operating room. Fellow patients and I were present to provide Cujo with a gift on behalf of the hospital. Afterwards I got the opportunity to meet him for the first time and had him autograph my jersey.

When a new round of CT scans came back on August 21, 2002, the results were very positive: my tumour had decreased in size by a whopping two millimetres! This may not sound like much, but in fact was quite a significant shrinkage. This now created another window of opportunity. The plan was now to undergo two more rounds of chemo, then attempt to remove only the tumour, thus sparing my eye. The doctors felt that the tumour could now be contained in a capsulated form, and therefore allow it to be removed without the more radical surgery. This was great news and made me ecstatic. I had gained five pounds, was about to be a guest at my old friend Johnny Bower's goalie school, and had begun playing organized basketball. I was feeling great!

With anticipation and high hopes for my upcoming surgery, my next two chemotherapy sessions flew by. Upon completion of my thirteenth and final round, I felt an overwhelming sense of victory. I had gone the distance, like Muhammad Ali's thirteen-round fight against Joe Frazier better known as the "Thrilla in Manilla." Ali had drawn up all he had left in him to defeat Frazier and claim the crown as heavyweight champion of the world. For me, it was like I was Ali and my cancer was Frazier.

Eleven years before, I was born on Thanksgiving Day. In 2002, my birthday landed on Thanksgiving again and it was very timely. It had been another challenging year, but the worst appeared to be over. With my surgery only ten days away, I had so much to be thankful for and I was not taking anything for granted. My parents, grandparents and brothers who missed school that day were on hand to witness what could be the culmination of my battle. We arrived early that morning. I checked in, changed into my garments and awaited my turn. I was led into the procedure room. Fearlessly, I jumped onto the operating table, felt the effects of my watermelon anesthesia, and I drifted off to sleep. A few hours later and with much uneasiness, my parents spotted Dr. Hurwitz from afar. From what I was told, my surgeon thought the surgery was such a success that he was practically doing cartwheels while approaching my family in the waiting room. He repeated enthusiastically, "I got it all! I got it all!" He had felt that he had gotten clear margins and had removed the entire tumour without damaging my eye. Meanwhile back in the recovery room, I was resting peacefully. Upon awakening, my parents recall my first words were: "Did they take my eye?" In a few days, we were to receive the full pathology report and then, if the report was negative, the plan was to continue with a few more rounds of chemotherapy. I'd then proceed onto a three-month follow-up, which we were all excited about.

EIGHT
Radical Surgery

When I was first diagnosed, Dr. Pashby referred to my cancer as "sinister." A year and a half later I faced the word "radical."

As we waited for the pathology report, one evening my dad knocked on my bedroom door before opening it. I was sitting at my desk. In a calm voice he said, "Andrew, there is a chance that they may have to remove your eye." I glanced up at him, but gave no response, continuing what I was working on. I later went downstairs and did something unusual. While sitting on the couch watching television, my dad vividly recalls me placing my hand up and over my left eye in simulation of what it would be like to live without it.

A week after the surgery Dr. Malkin called with the results of the pathology report. He explained it to my parents who were huddled around the telephone, "Rhabdomyosarcoma cells were present right up to the edge of the tissue removed and therefore there must be some remaining." He continued, "Relapsing so soon after his initial protocol of radiation and chemo and to still have cancer cells after the last six months of chemo means we now have to take more drastic measures to ensure the cancer doesn't spread."

My last resort was to undergo the radical exenteration surgery which would include the removal of my left eye and all the tissue in my orbital region. Prior to confirming the go-ahead with the surgery, my oncologist asked my parents as a part of his obligation to his oath, "Are you sure, as you also have to consider Andrew's quality of life." This must have been a very difficult question for my parents to face, but thankfully, they proceeded with the surgery option. When the surgery was confirmed, my dad once again had the task of breaking the news to me. After he told me, he recalls I put my head down while a few tears trickled down my cheeks before I headed off to bed. I came to accept my new fate and the procedure which lay ahead.

In preparation for living the rest of my days with one eye, Dr. Malkin thought it would be a good idea for me to visit the only other child in SickKids history to successfully undergo the surgery. His name was Spencer Matheson. It was his family I had seen years before on the first SickKids telethon I watched. Spencer had undergone the exenteration surgery a few years prior, so we travelled to St. Catharines, Ontario which was about an hour and a half away from where we lived. The Mathesons were a very warm and inviting family. Spencer's parents answered a lot of my parents' questions while seated in the family room. Spencer's brother also came out so say hi. He had had his leg amputated due to cancer, around the same time as Spencer's treatments. Spencer, my brother Justin, and I went outside to play basketball. I remember defending against Spencer very lightly in fear of hitting him in the eye, but he was fearless. He wore a pirate-like patch over his eye and was very comfortable with it. Afterwards, Spencer's parents called us back into the family room to show us what Spencer's orbital region looked like post-operation. As he removed his patch and his eye socket lay bare, I was taken aback a little by its hollowness but after a few minutes, I grew comfortable with it. Overall, it was a great experience and education for my family and me during our visit to the Mathesons' home. For a few years afterwards, our families remained in contact and the Matheson family became annual guests at our charity golf tournament. The last I heard, Spencer is doing well and is touring the world behind the controls of giant ships as a helmsman.

My surgeon, Dr. Hurwitz, was tasked with the role of performing the exenteration surgery. During one of my pre-surgery visits, he suggested that I should practise adjusting to living with one eye beforehand. So on our way home, my dad purchased an eye patch from the corner store that I wore around home for a few days. I practised reading, eating, watching television and even playing basketball, with the patch covering my left eye. The first night I wore the patch, I was sitting at the dinner table when one of my parents came home and was startled. Although I'd taken the patch for a few spins around the block, it was difficult getting used to and caused some dizziness.

With the biggest day of my life only a week away and my future uncertain, my dad decided to be proactive. He placed a call through to the president and CEO of Maple Leafs Sports and Entertainment, Richard Peddie. Miraculously his call went through and my dad told him all about my story, my upcoming surgery, and that I was a big fan. Mr. Peddie came through in amazing fashion: we were given courtside seats to watch the Toronto Raptors versus the Utah Jazz. Better yet, during the warm-up, I got to pass the ball to star power forward Antonio Davis while he was running side-to-side taking jump shots. About fifteen minutes before the game and while the players recessed into the dressing room, I was alone on the court taking shots as the fans entered into the arena. I received the opportunity to meet several more players including Vince Carter. Vince was injured at the time and was dressed in casual clothes when we approached him in the tunnel. Amazingly he remembered us from the last visit a year earlier. After the first quarter we were invited for a tour of the locker room. We entered and saw where the players hung out in a room with a large black couch and a fridge full of delicious Gatorade. We quickly glanced at the bathrooms which had sinks built to Goliath proportions. Next we went to the round room with each player's locker. I went straight to Vince's chair, sat down and slipped my foot into his sneaker. Unlike Cinderella, his size sixteen shoe didn't quite fit! During one play of the game there was a loose ball rolling in my direction. The Utah Jazz player dove to keep it inbound and his hand landed right by my feet. I was afraid I was going to spill my drink, as the ball got lodged under my chair. During one of the timeouts, a referee came over, asked me to stand up, and spun the basketball on my bald head a few times. That was very neat and overall was an unforgettable experience.

The next day we had tickets to a Toronto Maple Leafs game, and my dad worked his magic again. During the game, everyone seated in our section turned their heads and began to make some commotion. To our left was a woman accompanied by the Leafs mascot, Carlton the Bear, and Hall of Fame goalie and Leafs president, Ken Dryden. To my surprise, they were looking for me. My dad must have told them where we were sitting, as they called us out and into the hallway to speak briefly. We chatted a bit about hockey and my fight with cancer before snapping a picture and heading off.

I went into my surgery on a high.

November 19, 2002 was the day of my radical exenteration surgery. I was accompanied by my parents and my mom's father, Nonno Nicolo. As with every surgery, I checked into the allotted room on an empty stomach, was weighed in (at 37.4 kilograms), and changed into my hospital garments. This time I brought a goalie mask colouring book which featured all the goalies in the NHL and their different masks. I made good use of this book as the wait seemed to last a lifetime. Finally, we were called into another waiting room, down the hall. I remember this room was very large, empty, painted white and contained a few chairs in one corner of the room.

Before long, my surgeon, Dr. Hurwitz, arrived and wanted to speak to my parents and me before the operation. We followed him into a small room, which I remember being painted in a light colour and had a bed to my left. My parents sat to my right, while Dr. Hurwitz sat across from us with one leg crossed over the other.

The initial plans going into this morning were to remove the tumour and my eye, leaving behind my eyelids. From a cosmetic perspective, this route would have been less noticeable, as I would only require a glass eyeball. Famous actor Peter Falk, who is known for his role as "Columbo" and the multi-talented Sammy Davis Jr. both wore glass eyes. There was also the option of rebuilding the tissue in the area by removing it from another part of my body, along with possibly reattaching the muscles so I would one day be able to blink again.

The night prior to the surgery, however, Dr. Hurwitz said he couldn't sleep well while thinking of the negative possibilities of keeping my eyelids. He explained to us, "If we keep your lids, the cancer might return in them, as all it takes is one cancer cell. To make matters worse, the cancer could then easily spread to the other healthy lid." Now I don't know if it was this sudden news, or the threat of my life's most radical surgery only minutes away, but I began to weep. I think the severity of the situation finally hit me for the first time.

But we stood up, I hugged my parents and Nonno goodbye and then proceeded side by side with my surgeon into the operating room. As we entered, I noticed many people in white garments prepping the room. I made my way over to the operating table in the middle of the room and climbed up. A nurse first attached a device on my left index finger with a red light at the end, then came the anesthetic mask along with some suction-like attachments to my chest area. As watermelon anesthesia began to fill my nostrils, I prayed a short prayer. I opened both eyes for what would be one last time, taking in the ceiling before I drifted to sleep.

Years later my parents told me a story which impressed on them the overwhelming severity of the surgery I was having. While I was undergoing the surgery, my oncologist walked by my parents and stopped for a brief conversation. My parents nervously asked, "What if this surgery is unsuccessful?" Dr. Malkin replied: "If Andrew's cancer comes back, then there is nothing we can do for him." He later realized that, although this may have been the truth, his timing wasn't ideal, and he apologized.

A few hours later I regained consciousness. I was too weak to open my remaining eye and see my surroundings, but I could hear several faint voices in the room. I recognized the voices of my family and another voice which sounded like the father of a friend on my hockey team. A few hours later, I had enough strength to open my eye for a brief period to see my parents and brother Justin. I also felt a large patch-like item covering the entire left side of my face. Shortly after, Justin approached my bed and asked, "Hey Ange, you want to play Crazy Eights?" I nodded as he dealt the game and pulled a chair over to the left side of my bed. But after a few hands, I was too weak and drowsy to sit on a slight incline and even look at my own cards. In order to finish the game, he verbally recited the cards I was holding.

I had not attempted to open my left eye yet. I thought that, by some miracle, if I tried at the right time, I would still be able to see out of it. But once I finally tried to open it, I realized there was nothing left to open, I would now live the rest of my days with one eye.

As a few hours passed, I quickly began to regain my strength which was approaching normal levels. In fact, my doctors and nurses were amazed that I required no pain medicine. The only pain I was in was the agony of being trapped in a hospital room. More than anything in the world, I wanted to be at home resting on my couch or in my own bed.

We soon found out that only twenty-four hours after the operation, I was given the option of being discharged. When I heard this, I had practically packed my bags and was ready to leave. But, my parents turned down the opportunity, electing for me to stay another day. Their reasoning, I would find out later, was that they thought it was just too early to be discharged and that, if a problem were to arise, the hospital would be the best place to be. They also tricked me into thinking that Vince Carter was coming to visit me. I remember jumping out of my bed and onto my feet, grabbing my IV as my dad asked, "Where are you going?" I responded while glancing to my left at them, "I'm going to use the bathroom, then I'm going to punch you both out!" I had a lot of emotion building up in me after the surgery and the loss of my eye, and I also really wanted to be at home.

The next twenty-four hours felt like an eternity but finally came to an end. As I changed into my clothes I felt stronger than ever, but it was some kind of a hospital policy that you have to leave in a wheelchair after surgery. I didn't understand at first as the surgery was to my face not my legs, but I had often enjoyed racing around in any unattended wheelchairs I found in the hospital, pretending I was Rick Hansen, so I was happy that I did get one last ride in a wheelchair, out of SickKids Hospital.

NINE
Road to Recovery

A few days into my recovery, Dr. Malkin called with the results from my pathology report. The news was exceedingly positive. He said, "Andrew now has a one hundred percent chance of shutting out rhabdomyosarcoma cancer forever, although, he may require some more chemotherapy or the implantation of radiation seeds in his orbit." What great music this was to our ears, but could cancer really be behind me?

I stayed close to home in the first few days after my surgery but I experienced a tremendous amount of support from my school, my friends, family, and sports teams. One day the doorbell rang and it was my Italian teacher, Signora Romano, who had a large get-well card signed by most of the school. I watched her and my mom at the door, while I peeked from behind our kitchen wall. Apparently, she had my best friend, Chris Tarsitano, go class to class to gain support. That was very thoughtful. The next day the convener of my Mississauga basketball league dropped by for a visit. He brought with him a basketball signed by my entire team. He stayed for about an hour, telling us stories and wishing me a quick recovery.

Meanwhile, I seemed to be navigating my way around with ease with my newfound singular vision, or so I thought until I went over to the home of one of my good friends and hockey teammates, Daniel Agostini. Daniel belonged to another great family. We hit it off during practice one day after finding out that we had a lot in common, especially our interest in basketball. From then on, we always sat next to each other in the dressing room. On this occasion, we ended up in his basement where an old ping-pong table was set up. We decided to play for a bit, as I wanted to try my hand at the first sport since my surgery. He volleyed the tiny ball over to me slowly. What had once been a routine contact had become exceedingly difficult, as I failed to make contact with the ball. After a few more misses, I picked up a tennis racket nearby and attempted to continue, though with the same unsatisfactory results. I think we both feared that our hockey team would fail miserably if I started in goal.

However, over time and with much practice, I would recover. Today, I could probably use a spoon to make contact with a ping pong ball.

Sports injuries are quite common in the eye region, such as those incurred by hockey players Bryan Berard and Bernie Parent. My favourite X-Files actor, David Duchovny, also has little vision in one eye after a sports injury. Because of this, even prior to my surgery, my parents had gotten me into the habit of wearing protective goggles. With only one eye left, it became vital to protect it.

One week after walking out of the hospital, I laced up my favourite red and white Vince Carter Nike Shox and stepped back onto the court with my basketball team. I was number five and sported a white arm band on my left elbow (like Vince Carter wore), and my Kareem Abdul Jabaar goggles. Our first outing was a game, and although my first few shots sailed wide and my court awareness was altered, I did quite well. I made a few adjustments and finished the game with four points. Our team actually went on to win the championship that season, and my game improved beyond pre-surgery levels.

In the meantime, I was back on the ice, but not with my Vaughan Rangers team. Instead, I was training with Jamie Mcguire of Powerhouse Goalie School. My dad and I met Jamie prior to my surgery and he was eager to help me get back to game form. He was a great guy, a great goalie, and a very devoted coach. My very first day of training with him was at Sports Village Arena in the town of Maple. As I stepped on the ice and glided to centre, I noticed Jamie in goal, wearing an eye patch. He had actually gone that extra step to cover up one eye to simulate what it was like for me. Doing this allowed him to alter his training methods. We started out at the far end of the rink, throwing the puck back and forth as if we were playing a casual game of catch. This was to test out my depth perception, and surprisingly, I was throwing strikes. We then worked heavily on my glove hand, as with no left eye I had no vision of my left hand while in goalie stance. The solution was to hold my glove out a little farther forward in order for my right eye to capture it in peripheral vision. Next we worked on wrap-arounds and maintaining my vision of the puck when it was behind the net, as I had a new blind spot. The brilliant technique Jamie taught me was to turn completely sideways so I could see the opposing player through the net. I would then quickly maneuver to either side depending on where the player travelled. This was the core of the skills and techniques that Jamie taught me, which focused on adapting to playing with one eye.

The rest of that week consisted of various skills and drills useful to all goalies with the thirst to improve. By the end, I was a different player and person. Along with being a goalie instructor, Jamie is the coach of the Men's Canadian amputee hockey team and wants me to be their goalie one day. He even gave me the opportunity to meet a lot of the players and ceremonially drop the puck at one of the games. We kept in contact over the ensuing seasons and developed a mentor-protégé bond. One day he handed me a medallion of his which signified that he was one-year alcohol-free. I had never known, but he, too, was a survivor.

December 21st, exactly one month after leaving the hospital, I was back in the crease for my very first hockey game. I had only practiced once with the team, but I was ready. Word spread of my return and my story, so that morning I was featured on the front page of the *Toronto Sun* newspaper, the amateur sports weekly, and the *Vaughan Citizen*. My dad has always acted as my unofficial publicist and would remind me of it often. The game was also covered by Global TV's Molly Finlay.

The segment aired that evening as a "feel good Christmas story." Elliotte Friedman from Hockey Night in Canada also covered the event with Score TV. Before the game, the camera crew filmed me getting dressed, and my coach's pep talk. Even the Zamboni driver, Steve, displayed my jersey on the back of his seat as he flooded the ice. My team and I stepped on the ice to the sounds of much cheering from the crowd. In attendance that day were plenty of family, friends, and members of my medical team. Others in the arena wondered what all the commotion was about.

The game itself could not have gone better. The score was tied, one-all, when, with only minutes left in the third period, a player on the opposing Duffield Devils team stole the puck and skated ahead on a breakaway. He was all alone and skating in swiftly from my right. I heard the anticipation of the crowd as he elected to shoot to the top corner of the net. It was a fantastic shot soaring towards the back of the net... that is until, with lightning speed, I stuck up my glove and managed to capture it. Outstretched in a Statue of Liberty pose, I paused for a few seconds in awe of what I had just done. The crowd was ecstatic. The game was concluded in a one-all tie. It was a great win-win scenario for both teams. The referees came together after the game and called me to centre ice to present me with a donation to my Sick Kids fund in the amount of four thousand dollars; the referees in the association donated their payments for the day. Usually after a hockey game the opposing players don't see eye to eye, but this occasion was different. As I left the ice, both teams gathered around to cheer, along with the audience in the stands. Inside the dressing room, I was presented with the game puck and congratulated on a successful return.

After the game, my family returned home to find a crew from The Score TV waiting on our doorstep. They conducted a brief interview followed by a tour of my room. I showed them the memorabilia I had collected from the many professional athletes I had met or been inspired by. My room included items from Curtis Joseph, Vince Carter, Mike Weir, Arnold Palmer, Roger Neilson, and so many more. I went through each item on-camera and thought the whole interview was a cool experience.

Cancer fighters and survivorship is a universal brotherhood which I like to refer to as *cancerhood*. No matter where I travel, meeting a fellow survivor or someone in the midst of the battle always creates a feeling of comradeship. The great Roger Neilson heard about my story and decided to get in contact with us. Roger was a highly recognized NHL coach who coached for twenty-five years in the league and led his teams to various successful seasons. Roger and I shared a similar battle with cancer during the same time period. In 1999, Neilson was diagnosed with bone cancer, which spread to become skin cancer in 2001. It was during this time he reached out to me through a letter and sent me memorabilia from his team, the Ottawa Senators. Sadly, Roger passed away on June 21, 2003, only five days after his sixty-ninth birthday. He established a foundation in his name called Roger's House in Ottawa which supports children and their families with life-threatening illnesses.

My dad and I were introduced to retired NHL player and referee Paul Stewart. We met Paul, proud stage three colon-cancer survivor, at his hotel and rode with him as he prepared to referee a Toronto Maple Leafs game. Through Paul we got backstage access to the arena, were the first ones in the stands while he skated around hours before the game, and got access to the Leafs' dressing room. In the dressing room, I saw the Leafs goalie, Ed Belfour, sharpening his skates and saw Tie Domi at the door. It was a great game against the New York Rangers. Afterwards we went down to see Paul in the area where the Zamboni was stored and the nets were kept. He handed me a goalie stick which turned out to be Ed Belfour's from that very game. In a gold marker it said: "To Andrew, keep fighting hard." As a goalie myself, it was a gift to cherish. Before leaving, Paul gave me a very special referee uniform of his from the Stanley Cup finals. It was a very generous gift.

I certainly didn't allow my disability to slow me down. I kept moving forward and returned to doing everything I was doing pre-surgery, if not more. That season, my hockey team finished in third place. This was a great feat but paled in comparison to my own personal accomplishment. At the annual Vaughan Rangers organization banquet held at a banquet hall, each coach got a chance to go on stage to announce the award winners for their prospective teams. Among the options were most valuable, most sportsmanlike, most improved and most dedicated player awards. When the time came to announce the most dedicated, my coach began to say: "This year it was an easy decision. When you have a player who has gone through as much as this young man…" As Coach Rob continued, everyone in the room began to rise and clap as my name was called. I jumped out of my chair at the back of the room and walked up the narrow path towards the stage to accept my award.

TEN
Singular Vision

For several weeks following my exenteration surgery, my father took care of the cleaning of my orbital region. This involved him coming into my room early in the morning before work to clean and change my gauze bandage. Lying down and having my eye socket area cleaned gave me a very awkward sensation. I now lacked feeling in the area due to several nerves being removed in the process of removing the tumour. Because my dad had taken on the role of cleaning, and because of my reluctance to look, I still hadn't seen what my eye socket actually looked like. Finally, one day in my parents' bathroom, I glanced for the first time at what I will forever face in the mirror. My dad recalls me saying, "Dad, it doesn't look that bad." Despite the heavy swelling and colour at the time, I knew I could get used to it. I did, though, refrain from touching inside the area for quite some time.

Returning to the hospital, I had my first post-surgery CT scan. More good news followed, as all chemotherapy and radiation treatments would be suspended due to the excellent results of both the CT and my pathology reports. My next scan was scheduled in three months.

After the success of my surgery, the last item on my to-do list was to remove my port. For over a year it had served its purpose and, Lord willing, would never need to be accessed again. This culminating surgery was scheduled and performed successfully. For days after the surgery, I was in excruciating pain in my chest and upper arm area. The port had, in fact, grown to become a part of me and its departure left a void. I slowly rehabilitated with various stretches to get back to par. In the spot where the incision was made to insert the port is an inch-wide scar as a reminder.

I wore a white piece of gauze attached with a piece of tape across my orbital region for a long time following my surgery. After that, we experimented with a brown bandage-like patch for kids, multi-coloured eye patches with straps, and finally the classic black eye-patch made famous by pirates. We even experimented with different materials such as leather and cotton, and went to several different shops to see what would be the most comfortable and durable option.

Once my orbital area was completely healed, the hospital made us aware that I was eligible to receive a prosthetic eye. A prosthetic eye is composed in two parts: the ocular (eyeball) and the prosthetic (skin-like portion) into which the eye fits. We were referred to the highly sought-after Daphne Archibald for the ocular. My dad and I both attended the appointment where I sat upright in her chair while she very artistically painted on an eyeball canvas. Daphne matched my right eyeball to perfection. In less than an hour she created a perfect match, vein for vein, with the utmost detail, a process I would have to repeat every five years.

The second stage in getting my prosthetic completed brought us to Sunnybrook Hospital to meet David Morrison, an anaplastologist in the Craniofacial Prosthetic Unit. (Try saying that five times in a row!) David was another great addition to my medical team with skills which only a handful of people in North America are qualified to do. We spoke a lot during the week it took to create my prosthesis. David told us that he and his colleague had done some prosthetic work in film in the past, including a piece for the movie *The X-Men*. He also introduced me to an inspiring book about a one-eyed pilot who flew successfully during

World War II. The process to create the prosthetic was fascinating. It involved making a mould using a clay-like material that was poured into my orbit and then quickly hardened to form the shape of my orbit. Once the shape was accurate and the fit was right, David baked the prosthetic overnight. In the morning, out came a usable mould made out of silicone.

David's next step was to match my colour tone, which wasn't the easiest of tasks due to my Mediterranean skin type with many influences. To get it right, we made several trips outside to capture different rays of light on my face, making the prosthetic suitable for all occasions. David would occasionally call upon the feedback of his assistant, Wendy. Once the colours were perfected, he'd pencil in a faint eyebrow, eyelashes, and a birth mark or two to add some character.

The prosthetic was then fitted with the ocular, courtesy of Daphne, and was carefully glued into place using water-based adhesives. This new prosthetic provided me with an option if I decided not to wear my customary eye patch. (The next step in the world of prosthetics would be to undergo a surgical procedure to implant magnets into my orbital area. Magnets would also clip onto the back of the prosthetic, resulting in a quick insert and a more robust fit. It would save me time each day in cleaning, gluing and applying my eye assembly. After years on the waiting list, I was recently offered the opportunity to proceed with the surgery, but due to the recovery time and the additional surgery required, I decided to turn down the option for now.)

Of course, if you look close or long enough, you'll notice there is something odd about my eye, but the prosthetic, paired with the right pair of eyeglasses, makes it difficult for a passerby to notice any difference.

ELEVEN
Rewards and Scares

This summer came to an end with the second annual Charity Golf Classic raising over $40,000. It was followed by a successful three-month follow-up CT scan.

In September, I began grade seven along with a good friend from my hockey team who had just moved into the area. I showed Julian around the school, introduced him to lots of people, and we sat next to each other in class, but I was only going to be there for a week.

Beginning the second week of school, I was going on a very special trip. During my treatment, my grandparents had kept me motivated by telling me that once I had completed my treatment they would take me to Italy. (My older brother Justin is still jealous and asks my Nonna to take him all the time.) We travelled for seventeen days, also accompanied by my Uncle Johnny, my dad's youngest brother, on a tour arranged through my grandparents' church. We visited locations such as Rome, Venice, Florence, Sorrento, and, my favourite place of all, Capri. We visited the most popular tourist attractions and churches, ate some of the finest food, and created unforgettable memories. I got the chance to see where my Nonna was born and where she lived until she was thirteen. I met relatives I never knew I had. They were very nice people and very entrepreneurial. Closer to Rome, we stayed one night with another relative who owned a tennis club. He took me for a tour and I played a match on clay courts for the first time in my life.

Before we left Toronto, my dad had written a letter to the Vatican, informing them of my story and that we were about to visit. We received a ticket in return that allowed us to get close seats during one of the outdoor church services in St. Peter's Square. We were sitting to the far left of Pope John Paul II, immediately next to his silver "Pope Mobile." As I peeked through the windows, I saw a large, red, felt-like chair that that took up the entire back seat. Before I knew it, we were called to join the lineup of newly married couples who were getting to meet the Pope. The line went quickly and, when it was our turn, my Nonna said, "Please bless my grandson" to the Pope as he raised his hand to bless us. When I turned around I saw a thousand cameras flashing.

When I returned from Italy, the hockey season was about to begin and my entire team had moved up a league. We were now in Single A as the Vaughan Rangers. Every time I entered the rink kids would recognize me and tell their parents, "Look, there's Andrew." We had a great group of players and coaching staff that bonded like a family. This year we went all the way and won the Greater Toronto Hockey League and Toronto City championships. I think we only lost a handful of games. The season included my personal achievements of a less-than-two-goals-against average and eight shutouts. But before the end of the season, I had already made up my mind that I would hang up my goalie pads. My passion for the game was wearing away and I had developed a new passion for the game of basketball. Hockey had been an oasis during my battle with cancer, a focus I really needed to have and for which I am forever grateful. At times I wonder how far I might have gone if I had continued playing goalie. My dad thinks that, with my combination of skill and dedication, I would have made the NHL.

I went on to lead a successful basketball career, beginning by playing in Vaughan with players a year older than me, and then moving on to play in Thornhill, hometown of current NBA superstar Andrew Wiggins. I also led my elementary school team as captain, averaging eighteen points per game. We had a great season with Mr. Sisti as our coach. Our season was highlighted by a finals appearance in the Father Bressani Hearty Party tournament. My dad was always supportive of me no matter what sport I took on. Unlike most parents, he was at every game, practice, and even away tournaments. With my dad in the audience, I always wanted to play as well as possible. One day, he and I were playing catch in our backyard and we discovered that I could throw very hard and accurately. Dad suggested I try playing baseball, so I did. He signed me up to play for the Vaughan Vikings. I played one season as the alternate pitcher and had lots of fun.

November 19, 2004, was the second anniversary of my surgery and a crucial milestone for patients diagnosed with rhabdomyosarcoma. I would now graduate from a three- to a nine-month follow-up time frame. On a follow-up visit with my surgeon, Dr. Hurwitz noticed something out of the ordinary in my orbital area. A CT scan and MRI were quickly scheduled to determine the extent of the situation. Unluckily for me, I had just had braces put on a few months prior and an MRI is a giant magnetic device so I had no choice but to remove my braces, which resulted in starting my orthodontic protocol all over again. After the scans were completed, my family waited on pins and needles for the results. Thank God, the scans were negative and I remained cancer-free. This was just the first of several scares to come.

There was another scare during a period of about a month when I was experiencing cluster headaches that encompassed my entire head. I went to the doctors and eventually had to undergo an MRI—which was negative for cancer. The cause of these headaches was finally recognized. during a routine dental visit, when my dentist realized I needed some more serious work done and was shocked that I wasn't in pain. I asked, "Could this issue be causing the headaches I've been experiencing?" He replied, "It could very well be the cause as it could obstruct the air flow to the brain." That ended up being the solution to my headache problems. I also had another experience where I thought I felt some pressure on my right eye. After all the check-ups, it appeared to be nothing and either went away or was just in my mind. Better to be safe than sorry is what my parents always taught me.

Up to this point in my life, I had received several awards for what others were calling courage. I was now selected out of 151 nominees as one of twelve Ontario Junior Citizens of the year. It is a great achievement which is accompanied by an event every year organized by the Ontario Community Newspaper Association. I was nominated by my local paper, the *Vaughan Citizen*, which had featured me several times in the past. The two-day event was held in Toronto and began with a tour of the provincial Parliament building, including a private tour of the Lieutenant Governor's office. I remember that office vividly with its large red and yellow carpet with a crest in the entryway to the mahogany-coloured room. I bonded with the other recipients and their families over the two-day event, and we met some very inspirational people. The Junior Citizen award recipients ranged in age from eight to seventeen, and included seasoned volunteers, philanthropists, cancer survivors, and even a heroic shipwreck survivor.

The final day of the event climaxed with a gala which took place in the hotel's main hall. We were all dressed in our finest suits and dresses as we posed for pictures as a group. Afterward, the hall was filled as the twelve of us awaited our turn to be called up individually. My story was recounted while I entered the hall where hundreds of people were standing. As I approached the stage, I was greeted and handed a plaque by the Honourable James Bartleman, Lieutenant Governor of Ontario, whose office we had visited earlier that day. It was a great event and honour.

I also received the TVO Kids Agent of Change Award for 2004 and the Today's Parent Award, along with a feature in *Today's Parent* magazine and a wonderful gala.

One day during grade eight, I was seated at the dinner table when my dad broke the news that I was going to be blessed with a trip. I had no idea about this so I asked where I was going. When he said, "Well, it's undetermined but it could be Florida or Calgary," I knew what was going on: the Calgary Flames and the Tampa Bay Lighting were on the verge of making the Stanley Cup finals. We ended up receiving two tickets to Game Three of the finals in Calgary courtesy of the Children's Miracle Network. SickKids suggested me for this trip since they knew I was a sports enthusiast. My dad and I flew to Calgary. It was the first time I'd ever visited another province in Canada.

The trip was filled with unexpected blessings along the way, beginning at the airport. While getting ready to board, we ran into a family friend who worked for the airline. This lovely lady bumped us up to first class. That caused an amazing ripple effect, placing us in the same section as the Stanley Cup custodians who were also on their way to Calgary for the game. After we got off the plane, we received our baggage and went to find our driver. Just like in the movies, the driver was wearing a classy black outfit and holding up a sign that read "Mizzoni." Immediately after meeting him, we were ushered to a private room where it had been arranged for us to see and lift up the Stanley Cup. I remember it being very heavy, as I posed for a picture with it in both arms. Our driver had the best fare of his life as he, too, got to hold the Stanley Cup. For the next few hours he showed us Calgary's greatest sights. As we walked into the Saddledome, I was amazed at how friendly people were. The fans were electric, as a sea of red Calgary Flames jerseys filled the arena. When Calgary scored their first goal, a complete stranger gave me his giant Flames flag, and I ran up and down the aisle waving it from side to side. Calgary won that game, although they would go on to lose the series to Tampa Bay. The Flames never got the chance that I had to hold the Stanley Cup.

A month later, while nearing the end of grade eight, I was told to stay back in class for a few minutes during recess. Wondering if I had done something to get in trouble, I approached the desk of my teacher, Mrs. Chiarella. To my surprise, she told me that I had been chosen by my teachers to represent my classmates as the male valedictorian. I was happy, but I remember replying, "What about the male athlete award?" All throughout elementary school I had dreamed of winning the athletic award just like my father had before me. I knew I had to be in the running as the captain and star of the basketball team, co-captain of the volleyball team, and a ferocious defenseman on the soccer team. I also competed in cross-country and track and field as a high-jumper and relay runner. For that award, I would have to wait for graduation to find out, but I had to focus on writing my valedictorian speech as well as keeping the announcement a secret from my peers.

During our end-of-year school picnic at a nearby park, my friend Gino brought up the topic of who might win the male valedictorian. I tried to look away and focus my attention elsewhere as he said, "How about you, Andrew?" I responded, "Yeah right, I would never win that!" with a straight face as if I was Johnny Depp undercover in the film *Donnie Brasco*.

My dad assisted me in writing my speech as he did with most of our speeches. As a songwriter and musician, creativity seems to flow flawlessly for him. The night of our graduation I was called up accompanied by my female valedictorian classmate, Olivia. At the conclusion of our speeches we received a standing ovation from everyone in the hall.

Next up was the announcement of the male athlete award. Our librarian and coach, Mr. Villardo, began by saying, "We usually choose one person, but this year we decided to do things a little differently." I held my breath as he announced the first recipient to be Gaetano, one of my best friends and star of the track and field team. The next named recipient was Julian, my hockey teammate and neighbour, and star of the soccer team. Finally, Mr. Villardo announced my name. I jumped to my feet and pumped my fist, feeling very proud as I walked toward the podium. The three of us posed for a picture with Mr. Villardo, while holding our trophies. I wasn't done there, as I also received a Christian Life Award to top it off. I was so happy that it made the awkward first dance with my mom a breeze. That night I felt like Michael Jackson at the Grammys, leaving with all the hardware.

TWELVE
High School: Healthy But Not Cured

A ll kids are worried about fitting in when they start high school and I was no different. Leading up to my first day of high school at Holy Cross Secondary School where my brother and many of my friends went, I was a bit nervous. I had heard stories of kids getting bullied, thrown in lockers and more, although these turned out to be false. I remember looking down on the first day of school to find that my school uniform pants were hemmed way too short. My mom had had them hemmed for me as if they were suit pants, while everyone else wore them baggier. I don't think I ever wore that pair again, as I felt embarrassed to be walking around with pants so short that you could see my socks.

While probably every kid felt that way at the beginning of high school, for me, having been through my whole cancer journey, I so badly just wanted to be normal and have a normal life.

And as much as people had prepared me for every stage of my cancer treatments, no one really prepared me for life after cancer. I started high school feeling rebellious in lots of ways, and tired of things like fundraisers and the life where I was defined by cancer.

Not long ago I read the lyrics to a song from the play *Next to Normal* that made me think of my experience at this time. The lyrics reminded me that there are still emotional side effects that linger even when it looks like life has gone back to normal after cancer treatment is successfully finished.

What made high school fun was the people. All my friends from elementary school were there, along with many new people and especially all the beautiful girls I was meeting. Each morning we would gather by our lockers, line up on each side, and begin to push those who walked by like a mosh pit. Within the first few weeks of school I tried out for the junior boys basketball team and was one of two grade nines to make the team. It was coached by my gym teacher who was a very nice guy, but often put up a tough exterior. In the first semester I got a 72% average in my academic courses and was pretty happy with that.

My dad and I had been close but now that I was eager to move past my cancer experiences and be independent, my friends took on the importance my family once had. I butted heads with my dad a lot and didn't listen to his advice. All the grade nines maintained a tight-knit relationship and attended a lot of parties, and went to the local movie theatre together on the weekends. At the beginning of grade nine, as an athlete, I was disciplined when I noticed that both boys and girls were smoking cigarettes or marijuana, but one night I met up with one of my childhood friends who lived down the street, and decided to partake for the first time in a few "puffs" of marijuana. I did not know what I was doing or feel much effect at first, but my plans were to test it out one time then move forward.

But within months, that one night turned into every night of the week, which then turned into multiple times per day. We would usually get the product from my friend's older brother, meet at our neighbourhood park and then smoke and talk, and listen to music, or rap. We were heavily influenced by the hip-hop music we listened to, music that glamourized a gang mentality.

Then one day while outside my neighbourhood convenience store, a friend and I witnessed a man walking from the social club next door towards his brand new, shiny silver Lamborghini. He popped the hood which was in the front of the car, and removed a silver briefcase. My friend knew this man and that he sold drugs for a living. That moment ignited something in me.

I had had my first taste of running a business around age eleven when my brother Justin, my friend Joe, and I decided to wash cars to make money. We had called ourselves "AJJ's Car Wash," after the first initial in each of our names. After designing, printing and taping flyers about our services to people's mailboxes, we went door-knocking to solicit our services for five to ten dollars per wash. It turned into a successful business.

Now seeing the success of this drug dealer, I decided I would try my hand at selling drugs also, specifically marijuana. Word of mouth quickly spread along with my business. Before long, I was getting calls at all times of the day from an array of clients, some many times my age.

But as my sales and usage grew, everything else began a downward spiral. By grade ten, my grades had started to slip, as I neglected to even show up for some classes. My relationship with my family began to sour more, as I was often very angry and consistently rebellious. Grade ten culminated with me receiving an average in the fifty percent range and failing my least favourite subject of all, math. This meant that I had to attend summer school at my school for two weeks.

I went to summer school every day with a friend of mine, but although we were at the school, we never actually did go to class. Instead it was like a big party with people from all different schools having fun and getting high. Until one day when, during a rare time of actually entering the school, I was called into the principal's office where I found my mom. To make matters worse, I had just smoked outside, which I'm sure was noticeable. While I stared at the floor, the principal explained that I could still pass if I attended the rest of my classes. So that's what I decided to do: say goodbye to my friends outside getting high and buckle down to attend class. This resulted in me passing and getting the credit.

By now, I was buying and selling marijuana by the pound. I also tried growing it. A few friends and I stumbled upon a clubhouse at the conservation park in our area which was abandoned during the winter. We educated ourselves, prepared the room with aluminum foil on the walls and special lightbulbs and took a trip downtown to buy a starter kit and seeds. The seeds were bought at a very sketchy hut in the middle of the city. Once completed, we had an ingenious hideout which had a secret entry and a television. After a few days, the seeds started to sprout, stem, and began to grow little leaves. All was fine until the plants were left unattended during the Christmas holidays and they died. We were upset, but on the bright side, we had our own little hideout.

Meanwhile, I found out that someone wanted to "jump" me so I began carrying weapons with me wherever I went. This started another hobby: weapon collecting. I had an assortment of switchblades, throwing knives, metal bars, and even a samurai sword that split into two swords. My favourite weapon, though, was my BB gun. It was one of the best ones on the market and its pellets flew a whopping thousand feet per second. It came in a case, with a laser scope and a silencer. I eventually purchased the most lethal BB pellets I could find at an army store in Toronto's Kensington Market. In time, I had an arsenal of weapons that even James Bond would admire. Luckily, I never did get into a fight throughout high school, although thinking back, it's hard to believe. I did have my fair share of close calls though.

I did other foolish things during high school. I had a fixation with stealing. I went joyriding in my mom's car without a license. When students in grade nine started getting tattoos, I wanted to be one of the first to get one. I knew what I wanted – my slogan at the time was based both on my cancer experience and my love for hip-hop: "Back from tha dead." I planned on getting the tattoo across my back, but it would be too expensive so I got inked vertically on my right arm. For a few days at home, I wore a sweater to conceal the tattoo from my parents, but my brother must have told them and one day my dad said: "Let me see your arm!" He was not happy, and I left to stay at a friend's home for a few days. At school, all my friends thought it was cool. (I was able to rectify this mistake years later by getting it removed by laser, a process that took almost two years and was ten times more expensive and painful than the tattoo itself.)

During this phase of my life, I put my parents through hell as they would say. I fought with my brother and dad regularly and got kicked out of my family home some nights. Sometimes, I chose not to come home and stayed at a friend's house. Several times the police were called, and every time there were neighbours outside.

One day I had just come home from staying at my friend's house for a few days to hear that my dad was coming home to "discipline" me. After hearing this news, I took off through our back door, hopped the fence onto the main street behind our house, and didn't look back. I ended up walking to the community centre next to my house and stayed there for a while. I tried to sleep in the community centre, hiding from the janitor as he moved around cleaning the place.

When I got hungry, I headed to the convenience store a short walk away. With the few dollars I had on me, I bought a box of strawberry Pop Tarts and a bottle of chocolate milk. I was unsure of where to go next until I remembered that the conservation park next to my subdivision had little enclosures that were usually open. I eventually made it into the park safely as the ground beneath my feet changed from dirt to grass. I then walked to the first enclosed unit, a portable toilet. To my luck it was open. I shut the door behind me and sat down on the toilet seat. It was about the same size as a telephone booth. I was now safe and it was getting late but trying to fall asleep was challenging. With so much on my mind, all I did was sit, think, eat my Pop Tarts and drink my chocolate milk.

Several hours passed before I opened the bathroom door and saw the sun begin to rise. I walked back to the community centre, since I knew it was now open for the day. Exhausted, I fell asleep on the bench in the middle of the hallway on the second floor of the building. People were passing by and looking at me but I didn't care, until one stopped. It was my father. He drove me home and said that he had to inform the police that I had been found. I later heard that they had looked everywhere for me, including in the ravine in my area, and even using a helicopter.

This episode was the final straw for my parents. It sparked many psychologist and anger management visits for me. I began with a one-time visit back to SickKids with a social worker, a visit that did me no good whatsoever. Then I attended a group anger management series over the course of several months. Every week my dad would drive me there. We would go around the table, talking, with hopes of alleviating our anger. On the very first session, we arrived early and I assisted the teacher in making popcorn for the group. I thought to myself, *this ain't so bad.* Six of us were quietly seated around a boardroom table until I broke the ice. The teacher told us to write down three things that made us angry. As a class clown, I wrote "running out of weed." When my turn came to read our lists aloud, everyone laughed and followed suit in giving funny answers. During other sessions, we did such things as watch videos on anger and its causes. Slowly we were getting to the roots of our own anger. We even took walks outside during the summer.

Our teacher was a very nice lady and the attendees were young people from different walks of life. The only girl in the group was there because she used to get violent with her sister. There was a short cool-looking boy who had issues in his foster home, a tall boy who I didn't know much about but who always looked high, and a very quiet kid. On one of our walks around the building the quiet kid started punching the brick wall outside a pizza store until his hands were bleeding. I didn't know how effective this form of anger management was, but it was a fun journey nonetheless.

One night there was an altercation at home and I called the police. They came rushing over and separated me and my family. I sat outside on our porch where a younger male officer attempted to counsel me while his partner was inside with my parents. I was having none of it, sitting arms crossed. The most vivid part I remember was that he put his keys down on the little green table next to me and said, "These are my keys—now what would you do if I left them here?" I responded, "Well, if you weren't a cop, I would take them." He wasn't exactly happy with my response.

This episode ended with me being driven in the back of a police car down to the SickKids Hospital Emergency Room for a psychiatric evaluation. It was the first (and hopefully last) time I ever make that trip. The police officer waited with me until I was seen by a doctor. This led to me having to take one-on-one anger management sessions at a compound-like place called Blue Hills. I was given the option of living there and undergoing full-day treatments, but I turned that down and instead went to Blue Hills twice a week to sit one-on-one with another very nice counsellor. Each counselling room had a large video camera in a corner of the ceiling and a large two-way mirror on the wall, like you see in police interrogation rooms. I started to open up to this female counsellor about my past and my future plans, and she spoke of her experiences. She asked me about my drug dealing, and whether I was going to continue pursuing that. She told me that her son used to smoke weed and joked that when he returned home, he would eat everything in sight. After several sessions, it was decided that I no longer was required to attend.

Back at high school, I was seeing a child psychologist named Dr. G once or twice a week. She tried her best with a textbook approach, but I wasn't taking a liking to it. Soon I stopped attending my appointments, using the excuse that I didn't like her style and that she couldn't relate.

It wasn't until I got suspended one afternoon during my history class for having an altercation with my teacher that things began to change. During my suspension, my parents were called into a meeting with the principal, vice-principal, and a social worker by the name of James Fraser. Apparently, an immediate spark ignited between my dad and Mr. Fraser. James Fraser recalls that my dad put all his trust in him to help turn me around. My dad remembers thinking to himself, if anyone could do it, this guy could.

I had seen this cool-looking guy in the halls the odd time but didn't know who he was or what he did. We officially first met when Mr. Fraser came to my religion class and brought me to his guidance office. It turned out that Dr. G had been using Mr. Fraser's office the entire time. I began seeing Mr. Fraser twice a week and we would talk for hours on such topics as sports, school, and my past, which he would relate to his own past. The reassuring thing for me was that I now had someone who understood what I was going through, Mr. Fraser having gone through various battles of his own in life.

Over the ensuing months, we broke down the real cause of my anger and rebellion. After a traumatic battle with cancer as a child, I had built up repressed anger that I had to release. I began to realize that the hospital had treated me during my disease, but never prepared me for life after cancer.

Mr. Fraser gave it to me straight: "You and I are both minorities in the eyes of other people. I am a minority as a black man, and you as having a physical disability." As a child I hadn't seen things this way, but as I grew up I had begun to realize that the world is a very superficial place focused on outward appearance. And, although I looked different, deep down I just wanted to fit in so I did whatever it took to do so—including using and selling drugs.

One day Mr. Fraser asked, "What do you think you need to help build up confidence in yourself?" The first thing that came to my mind was the prosthetic eye option which I hadn't worn in years and had now outgrown. Mr. Fraser enthusiastically suggested that I work on getting a new eye if that was something that would build me up. The next day I had my parents call both Daphne Archibald and David Morrison's offices. Within a few months I had my new prosthetic made and was ready to show to the world. The first day of school with my prosthetic eye felt very strange since I had not told anyone that I was making the change. I remember sitting in religion class, doing group work and feeling eyes staring at me. But after that first day, I was fine and it did help boost my confidence.

Mr. Fraser also suggested that I should start putting on weight, both to help me personally and with sports. I had always worked out to a certain degree, but I was still very thin thanks to my genetics. I remember sitting in co-op class and writing down my goal to reach 150 pounds from my current 130. Mr. Fraser's advice was to eat all the time. I started eating six to eight meals per day, working out heavily, and taking vitamins and supplements. Often during class, I would ask to go to the bathroom and come back five minutes later with a chicken burger. Toward the end of grade eleven, I had passed my target of being 150 pounds and was now over 180. I was looking great and my confidence was at an all-time high.

James Fraser had been born in Halifax, Nova Scotia to James and Cora Fraser. It was there that his parents ingrained in him the faith and qualities he needed to make it through the obstacles life would throw his way. One of those qualities that James exudes is respect for others. He learned this through his father, who served in the Canadian Forces for more than thirty-four years and achieved the rank of Command Chief Warrant Officer. He also learned through the help of his mother who served as the foundation of the Fraser family especially while his father was on tour. James reminded me of the respect that is owed to others. One day I was standing beside him when I received a call from my mom and decided to answer it like I'd done many times before, saying, "What do you want?" James quickly intervened. "Was that your mom? That's no way to talk to your mother—show some respect!" This wasn't what I wanted to hear at the time, but I knew he was right.

During this time I was still smoking and selling marijuana, and was threatened with expulsion on almost a weekly basis, but despite a few incidents, the teachers and guidance counsellors saw that I was getting back on the right track. My grades even began to improve back to grade-nine levels. In an effort to remove me from the school environment, I was granted the opportunity to take a four-credit cooperative educational experience in a workplace of my choice. Only one year earlier, my parents had been blessed with the opportunity to open up a Tim Hortons franchise, so I elected to conduct my co-op with them.

One night during grade eleven, a few of my friends and I had gathered at my friend Dean's house. Since elementary school, Dean had had a passion for music and rapping. Now he had a little home studio set up in his bedroom, so the four of us decided to freestyle. I had been practising before, but not to my friend's knowledge. When it was my turn, I closed my eye, grabbed the microphone and delivered lyrics and a flow that shocked my friends. This was the beginning of M.I.C. which is an acronym for Musically Inclined Creations and the name of our group. I called myself "Heat" after my fetish for carrying weapons, or "packing heat." We began recording our first mixtape after school. The album was called "Lyrical Assassination" and was composed of seventeen original songs. We later sold the mixtape at school and performed during talent night. It was my very first time performing in front of a large audience, but I loved it. Our whole lives became a big performance as we would freestyle with friends at the local park and at parties, along with recording hours of material on the weekends.

Dean and I recorded a professional studio album at Velvet Sound Studios in Port Credit, the studio where my dad had recorded years earlier. For months we would go several nights each week after school. Before we knew it, we had a complete album featuring several successful artists, musicians and even two Juno award winners. Dean and I wrote all of the material and most of the music was provided by Mr. Fraser who happened to own a music management company. Upon completion of the album, we took the project to Metalworks Studio, the best studio in Canada, to get it mastered.

I arranged a professional photo session in various places across the city, including inside a Lamborghini dealership. Using these images, we were able to build our website and start promoting ourselves.

Next we tackled the packaging, working with a company my dad had used years prior. I worked hand in hand with their designer until the project was complete. One day I had a vision of what the perfect album cover would look like and bounced it off Dean and Mr. Fraser. They concurred and it turned out even better than expected. After flirting with a few names, the album was titled "The Hope." We tag-lined our music "hip hop with a conscience," as we featured several positive and uplifting songs. The cover contained a picture of us in white tuxedos, surrounded by clouds with gold gates opened in front of us. We were very happy with the finished product.

We hired a promotional company to promote us to radio and into the industry. We were represented at the world's largest music conference in France. We also began performing at several venues. We put on action-packed shows wherever we went, complete with a DJ, special guest performers and musicians, clothing changes and creative on-stage antics. Our album release party was held at the famous Reverb Nightclub where we stunned the crowd of hundreds. We went on to win several Battle of the Bands competitions, winning such prizes as a music video production. We even appeared at The Docks nightclub in Toronto where many famous artists have performed. I thoroughly enjoyed performing, especially hearing all the girls that screamed when I removed my shirt on stage. At every show and with every album sale, we made a point of accepting donations and donating a portion of our proceeds to SickKids Hospital.

Our musical aspirations also led us to be introduced to several influential people. We were introduced to the very successful entrepreneur and philanthropist, David Singh at a Career Day put on by another high school. I was invited through Mr. Fraser to attend along with busloads of students from various schools. As we waited to exit our bus, I saw a beautiful blue Aston Martin pull into the parking lot. Out stepped an impeccably dressed man in a blue pinstriped suit. I said to myself, *wow, who is this guy?* He was the last person to speak. He came to this country with twenty-two dollars in his pocket and eventually founded Fortune Financial Management. Fortune was named one of Canada's Top 50 Best Managed Private Companies. He also co-founded the Infinity Group of Mutual Funds and sold both companies for a whopping eighty-eight million dollars.

We wondered if Mr. Singh was into helping out the next generation and would be interested in supporting our music project. Mr. Fraser emailed his office, mentioning my inspirational journey, and we received a very positive response. When we met with him, we ran through our entire presentation with him and provided him with our demo tape. He asked us one vital question, "Are you looking for an investor, or a donation of whatever I can afford to give you?" Without much thought, we blurted out, "An investment." Unfortunately, Mr. Singh decided to not pursue our investment opportunity, but we did secure the funding from Dean's uncle to complete the album and promote it to the industry.

We never did fulfill all our musical aspirations, but it was a great experience and acted as a productive focus which kept me out of trouble the same way hockey helped keep my mind off of fighting cancer.

By grade twelve, I had continued my ascent. One day in a friend's basement, I decided to pass up on the opportunity to smoke and it was like flipping a switch: I have never smoked marijuana again in my life. I've had many opportunities and have even rolled up joints for friends who were incapable, but I never have looked back. I also stopped selling marijuana, was exercising every day, and was doing well in class. Believe it or not, I achieved an average of over 80 percent in my classes during grade twelve and made the honour roll. I also became the captain of the Holy Cross Hawks basketball team and Mr. Fraser became the coach. I began reading for leisure as well to add to the transformation.

One evening while walking with my friends down the street, out of the blue, Dean asked us if we wanted to attend church with him on Sunday. We agreed and went to the church my family had attended occasionally for years, St. Margaret Mary Catholic Church. This sparked something in me and I began attending every Sunday afterward and even started bringing other friends to church. I sat on the balcony at the rear of the church directly next to the choir. I was asked to join the choir several times but I thought that was a bad idea since I've been told my singing voice isn't the greatest (although I beg to differ!). I re-ignited an old tradition of going out for a big breakfast of eggs and bacon after church at a diner my grandparents took us to as kids. Who would have guessed that I would have been able to make a total 180-degree turn? (The staff in the guidance office at school later told me that they knew all along that there was something special in me, that they knew I was going to go on to achieve greatness.)

By the end of high school, the students in my grade had broken off into little cliques. I went to prom with a few friends, the only one dateless. All throughout high school, I had refrained from having a girlfriend. There were a few interested in me and I in them, but I was waiting for someone truly special with whom to dedicate my time. I attribute my late blooming back to my childhood battle with cancer. At the time when my peers were going through puberty and starting to notice the opposite sex, I was in a hospital. When I returned to school after my treatment, I noticed my friends starting to date, something I couldn't fathom at the time.

Our high school graduation was held at a local banquet hall on the same night as Michael Jackson's death. It was a great celebration and I was the recipient of a Christian Award which symbolized positive change in a student. At the climax of the gala, we all threw our hats up in the air to salute the conclusion of secondary school. I remember tossing my hat up and it coming straight back to me like a frisbee. We ended the night sharing a cigar and a bottle of champagne in my friend Gaetano's backyard as we prepared for the next chapter of our lives.

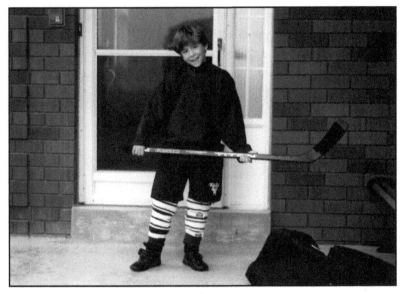

Excited for my first hockey season.

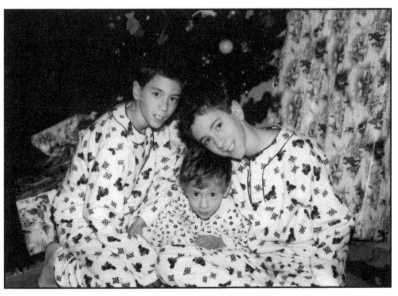

Me, and my brothers Lenny and Justin on Christmas morning.

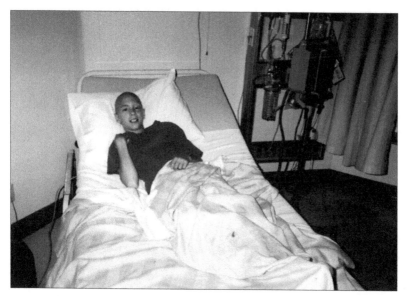

Undergoing my first round of chemotherapy at SickKids Hospital.

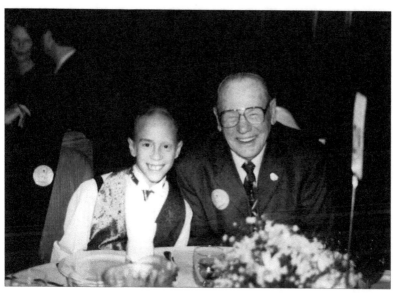

Two Great goalies. Me and Leafs legend Johnny Bower.

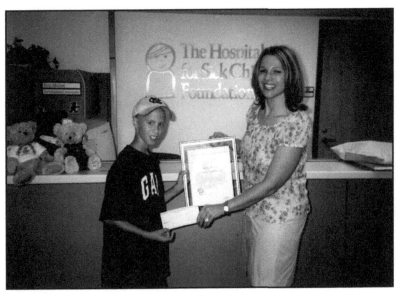

Cheque presentation to the SickKids Foundation's Eva Avramis.

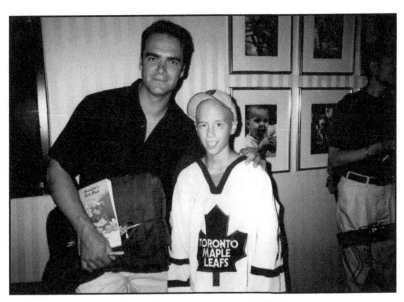

Me and Curtis Joseph at SickKids.

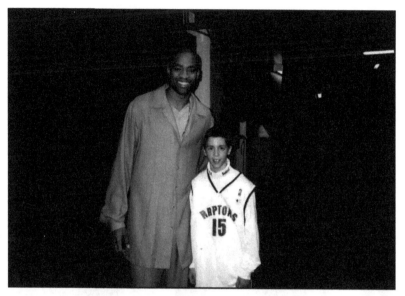

Vince Carter and me, the second meeting.

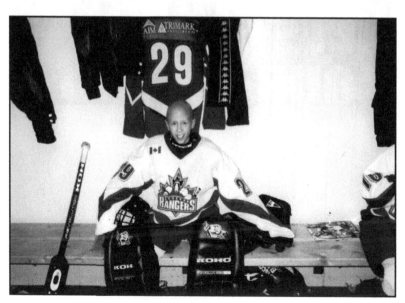

Focused before a big game.

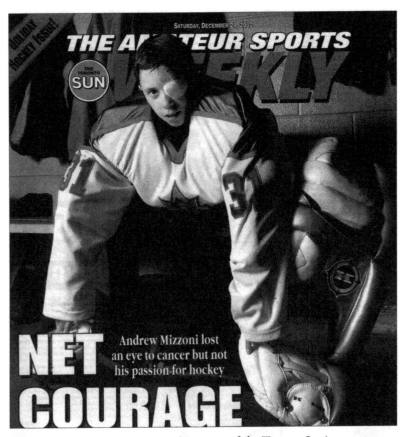

Net Courage cover (Courtesy of the Toronto Sun).

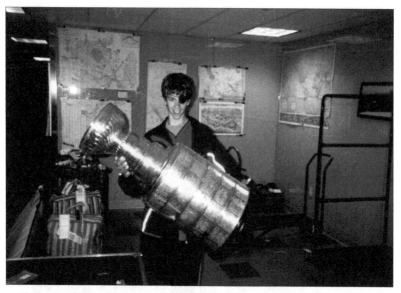

Champion! Holding the Stanley Cup, in the Calgary airport, on our way to watch the Stanley Cup Finals.

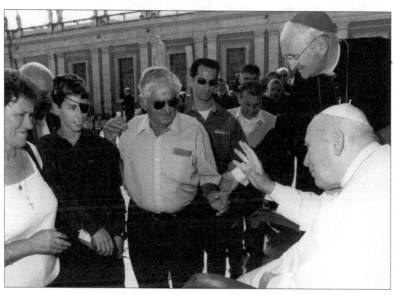

Nonna Esther, me, Grandpa John, and Uncle Johnny meet Pope John Paul II.

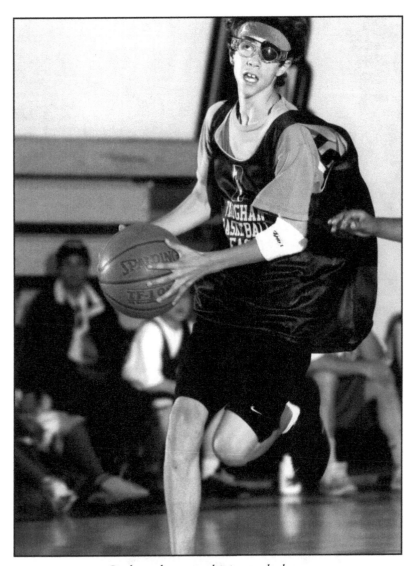

Back on the court, driving to the hoop.

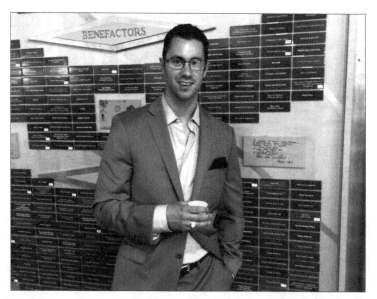

Enjoying an espresso at the donor celebration gala at SickKids Hospital.

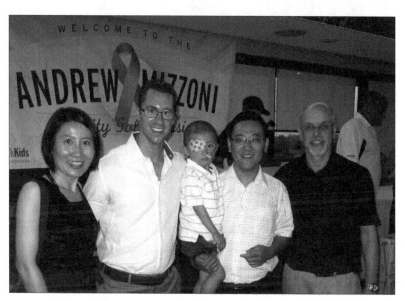

Regina, me, Wyatt and Jason, Dr. Malkin at the Andrew Mizzoni Charity Golf Classic.

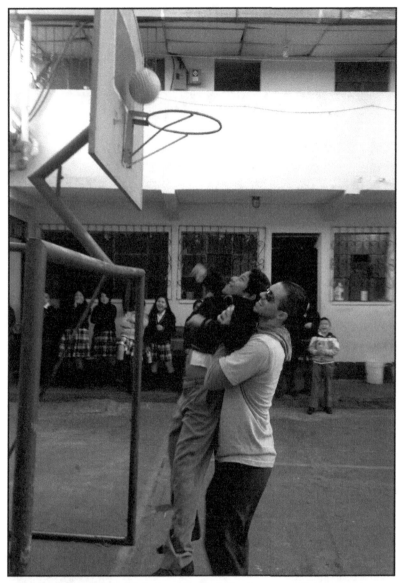

Playing basketball with kids in Guatemala during my first missions trip with NewLife Church.

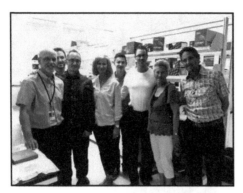

*Dr. Malkin, Justin, Dad, Mom, Lenny, me, Nonna, and Uncle Danny in
Dr. Malkin's new research lab.*

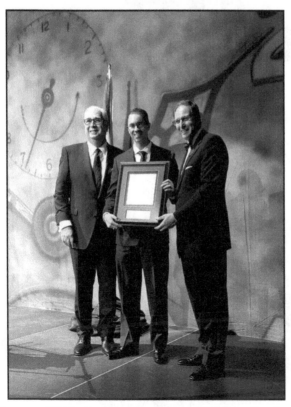

*Marc Caira and Eddie Burello—President of CIBPA—handing me the
Next Generation Award.*

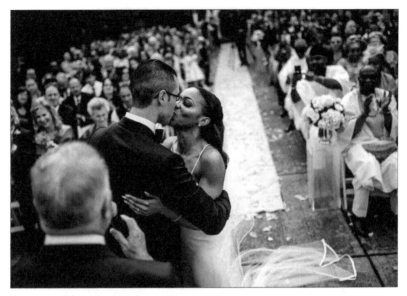

Our wedding day, June 4th 2017.

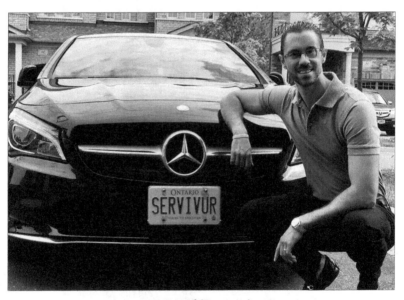

A Proud 'Servivur'.

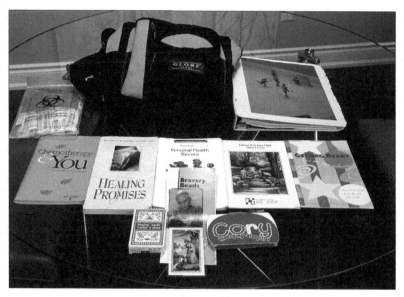

My hospital bag.

THIRTEEN
To College and Beyond

I had received a good taste of the business world and knew it was something I wanted to pursue. I decided to enroll at Seneca College for Business Administration: Entrepreneurship and Small Business. I decided to attend its newest campus in Markham which was smaller, recently renovated, and state-of-the-art compared to other colleges around.

Since I was studying business and wanted to make a good first impression, on my first day I decided to wear a full suit to school. This launched a habit of suit-wearing which lasted for my entire college tenure. My classmates treated me as if I was a lot older than I actually was and professors looked at me as if I was one of their peers. I was offered the staff discount in the cafeteria. On one occasion, I was even hit on by a teacher.

College was a great experience for me. I met a great group of people who came from various walks of life, some of whom I still keep in touch with. I learned plenty of knowledge which was useful in my career afterward. I also achieved a 4.0 grade-point average.

But after successfully completing my first year of college, I decided to take on a new learning path: real estate. I quickly ordered my first course and got cramming. Night and day that summer I read, made notes and tested myself over and over. My favourite place to study was outside on my front porch where I wouldn't be disturbed by loud voices inside the house. I successfully passed my first exam and perfected my studying methods to pass the second and third exams as well. I was notified that I had passed my final exam right around my nineteenth birthday, making me one of the youngest in Ontario to become a licensed Realtor®. Shortly after becoming registered, I received a letter in the mail from the Premier of Ontario, congratulating me on my achievement at such a young age. I celebrated by purchasing a nice gold Esquire watch for myself.

I was the third generation of the Mizzoni family to have a career in real estate. My great-great-uncle James Mizzoni is a legend in Toronto. He first began selling real estate in the 1950s and eventually opened up his own brokerage called Mizzoni Realty. His company sold real estate and insurance. In 1976, James would become the president of the Toronto Real Estate Board. He also ran for politics in Toronto and was an influential member of the Italian-Canadian community. My dad's brother, Danny Mizzoni, has also led a very successful real estate career. After receiving his real estate license at age twenty-one, he quickly found his way into management. He currently is a partner in a real estate brokerage and manages the new home division for some of Canada's largest home builders. With such big shoes to fill, I began reading all the literature I could find on real estate.

I joined my Uncle Danny's real estate office which is called HomeLife/Metropark. From the moment I started working at the real estate office, I made friends easily. This was much in part due to other agents knowing my uncle, but me bringing coffee to every meeting didn't hurt. Since most agents were more than double my age, I latched on to a few people as mentors. The first was a gentleman by the name of Louie. We would often have lunch together, drink morning coffees, and go golfing on Fridays. He even allowed me the opportunity to take care of his established clientele when he went out of town. I was receptive to any lessons he had to teach me and, of course, I was amused by his

Rolodex of jokes. The next person I came close to was Tony. We started out having coffees and lunches together and then progressed to me being invited to family gatherings and culminated with making wine together

After a few months in the industry, I started developing a passion for the condominium market which is booming across Ontario. After my first year in the business, I did fairly well and received an award for the most productive rookie in our real estate office. In my second year, I put my entrepreneurial skills into action. I found a niche in the market for preconstruction condominiums. I worked together with a graphic designer to create a name, logo, slogan and website and eventually "New Condo Mart" was born. I joined forces with another agent named Concetta. On our first site together, we set the bar to the sky by selling over twenty condos in only one week. We followed that with a few other successful launches that year. The next year we would add another member to our team, Lou, who is one of the smartest and nicest people you could meet. Together we launched a similar project focused on low-rise developments and called it "New Home Boutique." We sold an astounding twenty-two homes in one day at our first release.

I did continue to pursue my degree through online and night classes. In October 2015, I graduated with honours from Seneca College's General Business program. Seneca College featured me in their quarterly publication with a picture of me in front of a four-million-dollar listing with the title: "There's no limitations on what I can do."

In 2011 at the age of nineteen and with only five-thousand dollars to my name, I decided to purchase my first piece of real estate. It was a one-bedroom condo in mid-town Toronto. I only had enough to put down for the first installment but thankfully ended up getting the remainder of the deposit one way or another. It took me a whole five minutes to decide if I wanted to buy and which unit I wanted. It literally takes me longer to buy a pair of socks these days than it does to buy real estate. I find this is a trait that characterizes most successful entrepreneurs: to trust their intuition and make a decision on the spot. I have to thank my history with cancer for having such a high-risk tolerance. This particular investment ended up being a very sound and successful one which paved the way for many more.

After three years in real estate, I decided to add other skills to my arsenal and learn the restaurant business. My parents had opened a second Tim Hortons restaurant six months previously and were planning to open more. They mentioned that it would be nice to have someone like me to help run operations. So, I approached my dad one day and the possibility became a reality. I had worked in the business on and off since they opened, beginning as a baker, doing storefront and acting as assistant manager while performing my co-op in high school. I was capable of multi-tasking and decided to make the shift while still attempting to sell real estate at the same level. I began by shadowing my dad and meeting a lot of the new staff. Within a few weeks I was invited to the regional conference in Ottawa and was inspired by the direction the company was heading. That February, I began training at Tim Hortons University. They offer a mandatory seven-week course for all franchisees and corporate staff. Owners may also choose to send their managers and general managers. We learned about coffee and culture, production, floor leadership, restaurant management, and leadership. We also went on day trips to the coffee plant to see the process from bean to cup, as well as to the production facility where all the baked goods are made. I had a great time and met some good people in the process. In the fall of 2014, our family opened up two more restaurants in our area for a total of four.

In 2011, I took the helm as president and tournament director of the Andrew Mizzoni Charity Golf Classic.

FOURTEEN
From a Sick Kid to a Healthy Man

Anyone who has been a long-term patient at SickKids Hospital goes through a graduation once they reach the age of eighteen. They say farewell to the clowns, children's books and video games, and graduate to another hospital. Upon my eighteenth birthday, I went from having an annual SickKids visit to a two-year follow-up protocol at Princess Margaret Hospital in Toronto. Thankfully I was blessed with the opportunity to see a friendly face: my former radiologist, Dr. Laperriere whose clinic is in The Gerry and Nancy Pencer Brain Tumour Centre. It is the largest brain tumour centre in Canada, named after legendary Canadian entrepreneur Gerry Pencer who died after being diagnosed with a grade six glioblastoma brain tumour. What I like most about this centre is the framed boxing gloves hanging on the wall. They belonged to Mr. Pencer, and the legend goes that he wore them to a meeting while entering to the *Rocky* theme song to show that he was a fighter. How's that for inspiration!

In 2013, Dr. Malkin got in touch with me to see if I would be willing to speak with a child who had been diagnosed with the same cancer that I had had. I graciously accepted the opportunity along with my parents to pay forward the experience we received from the Matheson family ten years prior. The child is an adorable three-year-old with very loving parents. We decided to meet at a very familiar place for everyone: SickKids Hospital. The parents had various questions for us about their son's future which was at risk, while the little boy showed no fear at all. They had moved to Canada just a few years before and were overwhelmed by the obstacles they were facing. There I was ten years after my surgery posing as model for what a good life you can lead with one eye. His parents felt that he would be able to handle it well, but they feared for his future. Would be he bullied? Would he be able to find a date? Get a job? These were some of the questions parading through their minds. When we left that day, the family felt much better regarding what the future had in store for their little boy.

A few months later, his surgery was scheduled. Dr. Malkin got in touch with me again to meet with the family for a second time. This time my parents and I invited them to our home. We had pizza, cake, coffee and showered the young boy with gifts. They had a few more questions for my parents specifically. The climax of our get-together occurred when I removed my prosthetic eye for them to see. This moment was so pivotal for their understanding, as I remember Spencer Matheson doing the same thing in his family room ten years earlier for me and my parents. The cycle was complete.

I am happy to say that the little boy went through the exenteration surgery successfully and is working his way back to good health after a few other diagnoses. Today, he is in remission and attends our charity golf tournament every year. This past year, it was so nice to see him running around as I glanced down below from the podium while delivering my speech to cap off the evening's festivities.

Every year on November 19—the anniversary of my success over cancer—or whenever I am in the downtown Toronto area, I like to stop by SickKids Hospital to reminisce. I think it's important to never forget about the road you've walked to get to the road you're on. I occasionally stop into the chapel to spend a few minutes and often see a friendly face or two along the way. And I do still race up the stairs every opportunity I get!

Over the years, I've been the recipient of many stares and ignorant comments as a result of wearing an eyepatch or a prosthetic eye. I've heard it all from pirate sounds ("Arrr!), people asking me to see what's behind my patch, and many asking if I've gotten into a fight. It's very common for children to notice that I look different and begin to stare before saying: "Daddy, Daddy, look at that guy's eye!" It puts me in a very awkward position, but I have grown used to it by now. The most recent incident happened in Collingwood while I was heading to the gym. The front desk employee saw me and said, "Getting ready for the costume party?" Without getting into further details, I simply said no, and carried on my way. Following behind me was my dad. After signing in with the same unit number, the employee asked: "Is that your son? What happened to his eye?" Dad told him a little about my story and then finished by simply saying, "Google him." After I finished my workout and passed by the front desk, the clerk congratulated me for all I have done. If there is a lesson to be learned here, it is to learn to see past what only your eyes can see, for each of us is created unique in God's image.

Throughout the years, my family have been guests at many events affiliated with SickKids Hospital. Often, when we are introducing ourselves to other guests, we ask about their connection to the hospital. Unfortunately, we often hear that the person on the other side of the table lost their child to cancer. There have been times where we were at a table where all the guests had lost a child, and we were the only ones who had beaten the disease. It really makes you feel thankful for your health. It brings tears to my eye and motivates me to continue to do more, not just for myself, but for all those children who lost their chance. That's much of my motivation today.

Over the years we've had the pleasure of inviting various children and their families from SickKids to our charity events. Two made a lasting impression. The first is a young girl I called "Robin Rocks." In 2004, after she experienced shortness of breath while playing soccer, her parents decided to take her to the hospital. They later were informed that Robin had been diagnosed with rhabdomyosarcoma and that it had, unfortunately, spread to her lungs, bones and bone marrow. Through

Dr. Malkin, Robin and her family attended our golf tournament in 2006 and had a great time. Sadly, only a few months later, my family broke the news to me that Robin had passed on October 25. I still recall the green bracelet my parents gave me which said "Robin Rocks," along with "Help beat childhood cancer."

The second notable person I would like to mention is Christopher Stephenson. Chris and his father, Glen, attended one of our first golf tournaments through their connection with Dr. Malkin. I remember first meeting them as they were looking out over the terrace at Kleinburg Golf Course. They had such an amazing time, which sparked the family's fundraising efforts shortly thereafter. Chris also had a very rare form of cancer. As the eldest of four brothers, Chris was a great golfer and had aspirations of becoming a firefighter like his father one day. Sadly those dreams never came true, as Chris passed away in 2004 after a tough battle. The Stephenson family has since rallied behind their son's memory and have raised hundreds of thousands of dollars towards worthy causes. Our families still attend each other's events every year and have established a family-like bond. One year at Chris's memorial golf tournament, I had been having a difficult time all day with my game. Chris's father, Glen, happened to be at this hole and came up to me, teed my ball up at the back of my stance and said, "Try this, Andrew." I hit the ball beautifully. It sailed on a perfect trajectory and landed only a few feet from the hole. I immediately turned around exuberantly and said, "Thanks, Uncle Glen!" That name has stuck ever since.

Another thing I must acknowledge is my country. Having the opportunity to live in such a great country like Canada and receive free health care is a blessing. If my family had lived elsewhere and was unable to pay for medical insurance, we would have had to sell everything to pay for the hospital bills which would have probably been in the high six-figure range. I remember one medicine I was taking cost twelve-hundred dollars a day.

FIFTEEN
Where I am Today

I was still attending church every Sunday and sitting next to the choir, but I started to feel that I should get more involved. I contacted the church and applied to be a lector and read the Scripture every Sunday during service. Shortly afterward, my best friend Josh began a one-year Christian program in London, Ontario. He was immersed in biblical readings and passed on to me much of the wisdom of the Bible. He eventually inspired me to pick up the Bible I had had in my night table since receiving it in grade nine, which I had never before opened. I started with the New Testament and began learning so much. I also started uncovering differences in the Bible from what my church was practising. I had been attending church for most of my life but I learned more in one week of reading the Bible than in a lifetime of attending church.

I started talking to a real estate co-worker I knew was a Christian. David told me all about his journey to faith, how his son is a pastor, and used to pastor at a church in Vaughan called NewLife. He then told me to talk with another co-worker named Frank who still attended that church. When I talked to Frank, he told me about his wife's miraculous journey back to good health. She had been very ill in the hospital, and the doctors had talked to him about her options, including pulling the plug. At that moment, Frank remembers everything around him going quiet as he had a sense of a presence with him and heard a voice telling him, "Not yet, Frank." His wife miraculously came back to life after that moment. Nurses, who had seen her in her poor state, visited her and called her "the miracle lady." Frank and his family were all baptized at NewLife.

I like the famous parable in which a man decides to wait out a storm saying, "If I'm in danger, then God will send a miracle to save me." Neighbours offer him space in their car, a man offers him a spot in a canoe, a helicopter drops him a ladder but he rejects their rescue, and drowns, only for God to say, "I sent you a car. I sent you a canoe. I sent you a motorboat. I sent you a helicopter. What more were you looking for?"

This story reminds me of my story of faith only instead of a car, canoe and motorboat, the Lord sent me a Josh, a David and a Frank, until I finally came to my senses and was open to change. I also see a connection to my faith and my experience with cancer, as I find that those who have been the weakest turn to God in their times of need. When Josh completed his program, we decided to attend NewLife Christian Church together.

From the moment we entered the front door, we saw a difference. People were so happy, friendly and the church included a lot more people around our age. Once the service began, I felt this presence that Frank was referring to, the Holy Spirit. As the amazing worship band began to play, I felt a sense of the Holy Spirit as I lifted my hands in praise and tears rolled down my cheek. From that moment on, I knew I was at home, and would have difficulty going back to my former church. I completed most of my remaining lector appearances with the passion I derived from my new home at NewLife Church, and then bowed out. Going to NewLife has changed my life. Along with being saved, I have been baptized, began Bible College courses, attended multiple mission trips overseas, met great like-minded friends, and even met the love of my life.

As I mentioned earlier, I was definitely a late bloomer when it came to having relationships with women. I'm very glad that I was led down this path of purity so I might one day give all I am to my wife. I used to tell my parents that I was waiting for the right woman, a godly woman. My dad used to joke and say, "I'm going to push so-and-so off a ladder when you're walking by, so you'll think she fell from heaven." I had a few crushes over the years, and often I would feel very nervous when talking to these women but ultimately I would be let down at some point. At one point in my life, I thought that perhaps marriage wasn't in the cards for me.

However, I kept affirming to myself that God had something greater planned for my life. I found a video on YouTube by Tony Robbins where he talked about how he had written out all the qualities he wanted in the ideal partner. Whenever he met someone, he would put them to the test against his list. He eventually came to his senses when he realized his long-time friend had every quality he wanted— and they are happily married today. I wrote a list of thirty-five qualities I wanted in a woman. On my list was everything from being a godly woman to having common interests in movies and music. I waited expectantly and kept praying and praying, and on November 1, 2014, the Lord answered my prayers.

Our church had organized a bowling trip and I had signed up at the last minute when I found out a friend was going. Uriel is a great brother and also the first person from the church who reached out to me. For months, I expressed to him my intentions of wanting to get to know more people from the church. On the day of the trip, I was unsure if I was even going to go, but I put on my favourite outfit and headed out the door. I said hello to those people I already knew and throughout the night made many new friendships.

At one point during the night, I saw a gorgeous woman in a black turtleneck walk across my bowling lane. Later, as I was walking towards the food, I saw the woman in the turtleneck again. I said, "Are you cold?" as she had her arms crossed as if she was. She let out a soft, "Yeah." I followed in true Romeo fashion with, "Are you going to eat some pizza?" She said, "I don't like pizza."

After bowling, some of my friends were going to our friend Betty's house to play games. I had previously turned down the same invitation and was still unsure, until I summoned up everything I had to say yes. When I arrived at Betty's basement apartment, everyone gathered around her table. One seat to my left was left empty for someone who had gone to pick up Chinese food. A few minutes later she arrived. It was the woman in the black turtleneck from the bowling alley! It turned out she doesn't eat much cheese, so she didn't eat the pizza and elected to order Chinese food instead. I found out her name was Ono.

We had such an amazing time, laughing, drinking, playing cards and learning about one another. Ono and I spoke about places we liked to travel, our favourite music (she was impressed that my music taste was so soulful for a white boy), and where we were from. She asked me to guess where she was from and I quickly blurted out "Jamaica!" but she was from Nigeria.

I had never been in a room with a bunch of friends who shared the same faith. The feeling was so warm and the connection to the beautiful woman to my left was so real. We played cards and I helped her along the way as she appeared to be playing things safely, while I showed her a different path. It worked out very well for her. At one-thirty, we hugged underneath the moonlight and headed home. When I got home, I thanked the Lord for all he had provided and slept peacefully. In the morning, I told my parents all about my evening and included that I had met a Nigerian woman and had had a very strong connection with her

Two weeks later, after continuing to get to know her more, I found my list of qualities in a partner from my desk and began checking off the items that applied to Ono. I couldn't believe that I had crossed almost all of them off except two that hadn't applied yet.

I had previously purchased two tickets when I found out Stevie Wonder was coming to Toronto. I asked Josh to go with me tentatively— unless I found a woman to go with, I had said jokingly. Now I had found a woman, and when I invited Ono, she was very excited and started counting down the days.

November 25, 2014 was our first date. At first I was a little nervous. I even prepared three questions to ask her. I made sure to wash my car before picking her up and made some hot water with lemon for her before I left my house, which I knew was her favourite drink. She came out of the house looking beautiful. Some family members wanted to see where she was going all dressed up and with whom.

On the way downtown, we told each other all about our life stories up to this point. We ate, sang and danced to the music of Stevie Wonder. It turned out my guidance counsellor, James Fraser, was sitting only a few rows away from us. After the show, we got into a conversation about our intentions. I told her that "I am looking for a wife, not a girlfriend," while she expressed her views on godly relationships. Our relationship has only evolved since. God always knows just what we need. If we wait expectantly He will deliver in His time, the best time of all. On June 4, 2017, Ono and I were married. She made me the luckiest man in the world!

My relationship with my family has never been better. My parents are still the same supportive, hardworking and loving caregivers I've always looked up to. We get together regularly and talk on a daily basis. My brother Lenny is maturing into a wise young man whom I like to think of as my protege and my brother Justin and I connect on a different level. He is always willing to go out of his way for people.

Eight years after graduating high school, I'm still there causing havoc, but, this time, it's as coach of the boys' basketball team. In 2013, Mr. Fraser approached me to see if I could assist him with coaching the boys. We've been coaching together ever since, both the boys' junior and senior teams. I love the game of basketball and being alongside my former guidance counsellor at my former high school.

In 2016, I became a real estate broker and, together with two colleagues, Frank and Steve, formed our own team called KGM Real Estate. We are expanding quickly, having added five new members to our team. We offer residential, commercial and investment real estate services. Also, thanks to following the actions of great mentors like my Uncle Danny, I now own multiple residential investment properties. Lately, I have been inspired to start investing in apartment buildings and to begin real estate developing in the Greater Toronto Area.

On my most recent visit to the hospital I was pleased to see my very first nurse from SickKids, Mary Stewart. Mary gave me a thorough explanation of what I have to look out for in the future as a result of the radiation and chemotherapy I had. The main concerns are future tumours growing in the brain caused by my radiation therapy and damage to my heart, ears and thyroid due to the chemotherapy. She ordered an MRI of my brain, a blood test to check my thyroid, a heart test also known as an "echo" and a hearing test. Sitting on the doctor's table, I asked Dr. Laperriere, "What else can I do to limit my chances of getting cancer in the future?" He said: "You're healthy as can be and you eat well. Just don't smoke." He said I could smoke the odd cigar with my friend Josh from time to time, but I think I'll have to tell Josh that I can't join him at the cigar lounge anymore; my health is no joke.

A healthy diet and exercise are essential elements of my life. Ever since high school, I have continued eating right and exercising at least four times per week. My gym routine changes from time to time to keep it interesting but it contains stretching, followed by weightlifting and then cardio and abdominals workouts. During the nicer weather, I enjoy going on runs outside and walks in the evening to help clear my mind. I started 2018 with completing the insane P90X routine. I also shop at a natural grocery store and eat organic and healthy food every chance I get. I am aware of the potential long-term side effects from my treatment, and this motivates me to do all I can to stay healthy and fend them off. I also play several leisure sports such as golf and basketball. They help me have fun, clear the mind, and get a good workout. My wife and I are proud season-ticket holders of the Toronto Raptors and enjoy an exciting game of basketball often. One of my favourite hobbies is reading. A couple times a month, Josh and I will hook up for breakfast and then hit up the used bookstore and walk away with a stack of books. I enjoy all types of books but business books, autobiographies and the self-help categories intrigue me the most. My collection contains so many books that I should start issuing library cards. I find reading is a great way to expand my horizons, broaden vocabulary and let my mind escape. Whatever phase I'm going through in life, I try to find a book written by someone who has already faced such a challenge. This way I can learn from their mistakes instead of duplicating them myself. I'm also big on listening to motivational audio first thing in the morning to inspire me throughout the day.

My family's fundraising efforts for cancer research have now been ongoing for seventeen years. We've put on some great events and have contributed greatly to cancer research at SickKids and the world, helping to raise approximately $500,000 for SickKids. This is a large amount in itself, but what is amazing is that our funds have acted as the seed money to secure tens of millions of dollars in federal grants. Some of the work which started with our investment is recognized across the world. The first clinical trial sponsored by the Andrew Mizzoni Cancer Research Fund was up and running in 2015. It involves the drug tamoxifen, that is used to treat breast cancer, and can actually kill rhabdomyosarcoma cells. The protocol, which is led out of SickKids, includes partners from five other pediatric cancers centres in the United States. Dr. Malkin is also working with a colleague to target the protein dystrophin which is defective in children with rhabdomyosarcoma. They are running tests on zebrafish as I am writing. Another area of progress is from their massive DNA sequencing efforts. Instead of every kid getting the exact same drugs, we are at the point where we can "personalize" their treatment – and hopefully avoid many of the side effects. Dr Malkin addressed the crowd at our latest fundraiser with these words, "I say this every year, and I am confident in saying it again this year: we *will* find a cure … soon. One day, I do hope that there will be no need to raise funds for rhabdomyosarcoma or childhood cancer research because the disease will be a thing of the past. Until then, however, we have our work cut out for us, my friends."

Conclusion

Mr. Fraser had a poster in his office with an Alice Morse Earle saying on it. It said, "Yesterday is History. Tomorrow is a Mystery. Today is a Gift, that's why it's called the Present!" I used to look at it throughout the many hours I spent in his office.

As I write this, I have just celebrated my 26th birthday surrounded by family and friends. I feel I've already been blessed with enough experiences for a lifetime. I'm confident that anyone without faith in God should read my story and walk away with a renewed outlook on life. Just the slightest change in any direction may have altered my life forever and even my existence today. But, I know the Lord was directing my path and instructed the right people to appear as His agents.

I thank God that I was diagnosed during the time I was, and not later on in life. Being diagnosed as a child was a blessing, as I didn't pay attention to the odds and percentages that I would have had I been diagnosed today. My indifference to my protocol was key, and all I focused on was regaining my old life of being a playful child.

I missed a lot during my childhood years, which is why I try to keep that child in me alive and well today. I love hanging around kids, especially my nephew Manny, and enjoy spoiling them with toys. I think it's very important to always stay young at heart as we grow older.

My motivation in life is all those children who were suffering then and now down the halls of SickKids Hospital and all the other children's wings around the world. I hope my story provides hope to millions of them and their families and encourages them to share their journeys. There is hope at the end of the hallway. That is why I wrote this. This was my journey to become a survivor.

Helpful Links

http://eyewiki.aao.org/Rhabdomyosarcoma

http://cancer.about.com/od/historyofcancer/a/cancerhistory.htm

http://www.cancer.org/cancer/cancerbasics/thehistoryofcancer/index?sitearea

http://www.nlm.nih.gov/medlineplus/ency/article/003833.htm

http://www.cancer.org/cancer/cancerbasics/thehistoryofcancer/the-history-of-cancer-cancer-treatment-chemo

https://www.cancer.gov/about-cancer/treatment/types/radiation-therapy/radiation-fact-sheet

About the Author

Andrew Mizzoni is a childhood cancer survivor and philanthropist who has raised over half a million dollars for pediatric cancer research. Diagnosed with cancer when he was only nine years old, Andrew Mizzoni overcame the illness twice. He bravely accepted his treatments, surgeries, and the loss of his left eye with wisdom and maturity beyond his years. Andrew's story has not gone unnoticed: his story has been published in various publications across North America. He has received many awards and honours for his courage and fundraising efforts, including being named the Ontario Junior Citizen of the Year, *Today's Parent* magazine's Our Heroes winner, Agent of Change recipient and the recipient of the Next Generation award by the Canadian Italian Business and Professionals Association. Today Andrew has a successful real estate business and continues to inspire people with his positive energy. When he is not working, Andrew enjoys spending time with his wife, reading, athletics, travelling, movies, and hosting family and friends.

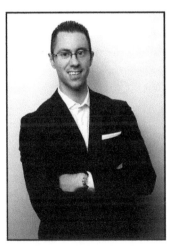

Find Andrew at AndrewMizzoni.com.